# Chronic Illness, Vulnerability Social Work

While the body has recently assumed greater sociological significance, there has been less engagement in social work and social care on the bodily experience of health, illness and disease. This innovative volume redresses the balance by exploring chronic illness and social work, through the specific lens of autoimmunity, engaging in wider debates around vulnerability, resistance and the lived experience of ongoing ill-health.

Moving beyond existing conceptualisations of vulnerability as an issue of mental distress, ageing, child protection or poverty, Price and Walker demonstrate the role that social work has to play in actively engaging the physical body, rather than working around and through it. The book focuses on autoimmune conditions such as lupus, multiple sclerosis, rheumatoid arthritis and scleroderma. Conditions like these allow for an exploration of the materiality of illness that exacerbates social and economic vulnerability and may precipitate personal and social crises, requiring a variety of interventions and support. The risks and challenges associated with chronic illness include disruptions to a sense of self and identity, altered relationships and the renegotiation of roles and responsibilities in a variety of relationships, in addition to an economic impact, with the potential for disruption to employment status and financial insecurity.

This text opens up a range of debates around some of the central concerns of the social work profession, including vulnerability, ill-health and independence. It will be of interest to scholars and students of social work, nursing, disability studies, medicine and the social sciences.

**Liz Price** is Senior Lecturer in Social Work at the University of Hull, UK. She is a registered social worker and her research interests currently include the lived experience of chronic illness, sexualities and dementia, the sociology of dental intervention and the use of music as a therapeutic tool.

**Liz Walker** is Reader in Social Work at the University of Hull, UK. She is a registered social worker and medical sociologist. Her research interests are in HIV/AIDS, the sociology of chronic illness and marginal masculinities.

# Routledge Advances in Social Work

## New titles

**Analysing Social Work Communication**
Discourse in practice
*Edited by*
*Christopher Hall, Kirsi Juhila, Maureen Matarese and Carolus van Nijnatten*

**Feminisms in Social Work Research**
Promise and possibilities for justice-based knowledge
*Edited by*
*Stéphanie Wahab, Ben Anderson-Nathe and Christina Gringeri*

**Chronic Illness, Vulnerability and Social Work**
Autoimmunity and the contemporary disease experience
*Liz Price and Liz Walker*

## Forthcoming titles

**Social Work in a Global Context**
Issues and challenges
*Edited by*
*George Palattiyil, Dina Sidhva and Mono Chakrabarti*

**Contemporary Feminisms in Social Work Practice**
*Edited by*
*Nicole Moulding and Sarah Wendt*

**Domestic Violence Perpetrators**
Evidence-informed responses
*John Devaney, Anne Lazenbatt and Maurice Mahon*

# Chronic Illness, Vulnerability and Social Work

Autoimmunity and the contemporary disease experience

**Liz Price and Liz Walker**

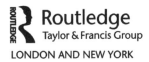
Routledge
Taylor & Francis Group

LONDON AND NEW YORK

First published 2015
by Routledge
2 Park Square, Milton Park, Abingdon, Oxon OX14 4RN

and by Routledge
711 Third Avenue, New York, NY 10017

First issued in paperback 2017

*Routledge is an imprint of the Taylor & Francis Group, an informa business*

*British Library Cataloguing in Publication Data*
A catalogue record for this book is available from the British Library

*Library of Congress Cataloguing in Publication data*
Price, Liz (Senior lecturer in social work), author.
  Chronic illness, vulnerability and social work : autoimmunity and the contemporary disease experience / written by Liz Price and Liz Walker.
    p. ; cm. – (Routledge advances in social work)
  Includes bibliographical references and index.
  I. Walker, Liz (Reader in social work), author. II. Title. III. Series: Routledge advances in social work.
  [DNLM: 1. Chronic Disease–psychology. 2. Social Work. 3. Autoimmune Diseases–psychology. 4. Body Image. 5. Self Concept. WT 30]
  RB127.5.C48
  616'.047–dc23
  2014044141

ISBN 13: 978-1-138-49455-8 (pbk)
ISBN 13: 978-0-415-64353-5 (hbk)

Typeset in Garamond
by Out of House Publishing

For Rob Juson

# Contents

# Figures

# Acknowledgements

In writing this book, we have been fortunate to have enjoyed the support and encouragement of a great many people. We would like to thank, in particular, all those who have generously shared their stories with us. Some of their experiences are to be found in the chapters that follow and the artwork of Carole Chisholm and Lin-Marie Milner Brown, found in Chapter 4, helps to bring these experiences to life. We wish also to applaud their courage and tenacity in living with lupus, this most challenging of long-term illnesses. In doing so, we remember with great sadness those people we interviewed who have died with lupus while we have been writing about their lives. We are thinking, in particular, of Val Wilson, who provided such enthusiasm and support despite her own difficulties.

Thanks are also due to Chris Maker, director of Lupus UK, who facilitated our research and to both the charity and the University of Hull Faculty Strategic Support Fund for funding our original research.

Our colleagues in the School of Social Sciences at the University of Hull (and beyond) have been patient and often inspiring in providing an environment in which to explore and develop our ideas.

It is inevitable that there are unintended casualties of a project such as this and, at this point, we would like to apologise to Adrienne and Erin for what they may perceive to have been issues of profound parental intellectual absence and inattention.

Finally, and most importantly, we thank Rob Juson, without whose support and friendship the project as a whole would simply not have been possible. Rob is an inspiration and seemingly endless source of enthusiasm and energy (although we know that this may be at great cost to himself). We dedicate this book to him.

# Introduction

In the summer of 2008 I had accompanied a friend to a hospital appointment. As I waited for her, in a ubiquitous beige-coloured corridor, to complete her consultation, I idly leafed through a range of patient information leaflets that were displayed on the wall in front of me. One in particular generated something of a light bulb moment, describing, in remarkably concise detail, many of the seemingly inexplicable physical difficulties I myself had been experiencing for some time. The leaflet contained information on a condition called polymyalgia rheumatica and, having been unable to lift my arms above shoulder height and being similarly inept at rising comfortably from a chair for many months, this autoimmune condition, which causes pain, stiffness and inflammation in the muscles around the shoulders, neck and hips, might, I thought, provide some sort of explanation.

In the coming months, as the symptoms worsened and started to seriously impact upon everyday activities, I sought professional confirmation of my chance diagnostic discovery. This, although I was unaware of it at the time, was to be the start of a long and protracted journey into both a personal and professional illness experience. The diagnosis, was not, as it turned out, polymyalgia rheumatica, but suspected systemic lupus erythematosus (SLE or, more commonly, lupus), another of the many autoimmune conditions. This diagnosis itself, however, was set to shift and change (an experience reflected in many others' experiences in the coming pages) coming to rest (for now, at least), some six years later, in a diagnosis of another different, but similarly serious, systemic condition.

It was this experience that led me to my interest in other people's experiences and understandings of what it means to have an autoimmune condition. I wondered, selfishly, if my experience was unique or whether, in fact, the difficulties inherent in my own experience of autoimmunity were perhaps more common than I might imagine. Chance conversations with my friend and colleague, Liz Walker, confirmed that this commonality was, perhaps, to be found nearer to home that I had anticipated. At the same time that I had begun to be unwell, she too had begun a diagnostic journey to make sense of her own worsening health. We were, simultaneously, diagnosed with autoimmune conditions and it has been the joint articulations, both personal and professional, of our experiences that have led down a route of interest and enquiry that has generated a discursive exploration of the autoimmune experience and the various professional responses to it. First and foremost, then, this book is about the everyday lived experience of autoimmunity; an experience characterised by, and replete with, paradox, contradiction and the constancy of physical and psychological distress, a state captured by Andrews (2011: 25) in her autobiographical account of living with lupus:

> I am feeling unsettled, antsy and on edge. I cannot sleep, and I cannot focus.
>
> Cocooned in my blanket against the cold – I'm too hot. Feverish perhaps? I am sick. Nestled into my sickbed, surrounded by the trappings of comfort, I am uncomfortable. Incapacitated. I struggle to recall myself: I call to mind the relative comfort of illnesses past: my mother performing her nursing duties, offering me forbidden treats – a welcome day off school, day-time television, a film proffered as distraction from the seeming failure of my body. Then, there was a sense of security and consolation for I was experiencing nothing but a childhood illness; a normal, expected, anticipated sickness; a discomfort endured in order to build my immunity, to secure my body against a common pathogen as a means to protect and strengthen my future self. Recovery was foreseen, expected and enacted. Now, however, here, there is an apprehension, an apprehension of finality felt in my aching bones. An awareness perhaps of worse now to come... Now is worse for my illness is chronic, debilitating and uncanny, a strange, familiar, and yet 'unnatural' sickness. It is worse because my illness is not the result of a pathogen, a bacteria or a virus attacking my body, there is no (m)other who is threatening 'me'. My body is attacking itself. I am told that my own defences – my immune system – is, for reasons unknown, attacking that which it should be safeguarding. I am told my body's defensive efforts are enacting that which it should seek to avoid: a threat to the cohesion of the body. My illness, I am told, is autoimmune... I have systemic lupus erythematosus, or lupus. A name which has conjured a spectral wolfishness within me, manifesting as a terrifying series of repetitive attacks by a predator that turns out to be myself, myself as werewolf: foe as friend, other as self. In this sickbed there is no (m)other to protect and comfort me, I must comfort myself...

Our joint response to our own particular diagnoses was to ask the question 'how do other people make sense of this experience?' and our starting point for our exploration into the experience of autoimmunity was an empirical study focused on lupus.[1] This condition is experienced as skin rashes, photosensitivity, oral and nasal ulcers, serositis, arthritis, renal, neurological, haematological and immunological disorders (the American Rheumatological Association stipulates four symptom clusters are required to positively diagnose lupus). It predominantly affects women (seven to eight times more than men) and is more evident in certain ethnic groups (such as African-Americans). The incidence and prevalence of lupus is very difficult to determine, ranging from conservative estimates of 30,000 to a possible 50,000 (in the UK) and, in the US, 17–71 per 100,000 for Caucasian women to a high of 56–283 per 100,000, for African-American women (Manzi, 2001, cited in Miles, 2013: 24). Miles (2013: 24) further suggests that 'actual prevalence rates of lupus probably far exceed reported rates and researchers assume that mild cases of lupus are significantly underreported'.

The original research we undertook comprised a qualitative enquiry in which we asked people living with lupus to narrate their everyday understandings and experience of illness. We provided a thematic framework for these narratives that centred on the process of 'becoming ill'; people's encounters with the medical profession; the family, care and intimacy; encountering the 'everyday'; and the role of support networks. While this study comprises the foundation of our work for the book, it also generated a range of unanticipated questions and routes of enquiry that led us to understand the lived experience of lupus within the wider framework of the experience of living with autoimmunity more broadly. The data and the findings from this study constitute a very visible thread through each of the chapters in the book and provide a basis from which to explore and articulate the wider questions with which each chapter engages.

In each chapter, we purposefully foreground the voices of people with lupus, as they are all but silent in the existing social sciences and social work literature, as are the voices of the various practitioners who treat and support them (notable exceptions include Stockl, 2007; Mendelson, 2003, 2006, 2009; Miles, 2013). We would suggest that one of the reasons for this is the fact that lupus, like many other autoimmune conditions, is relatively rare and, thus, does not attract research, policy or public attention in ways that other conditions, such as cancer, dementia, heart disease, diabetes, etc., tend to do. Felstiner (2007) suggests that its gendered nature also accounts for its poor profile in the academic literature.

While this book is not a memoir or a personal account, given our own experience, we are inevitably and explicitly written into and refracted through both the narratives of our respondents and the theoretical frameworks we use to explicate and analyse them. Every interview and conversation has caused us to reflect on our own conditions, which, in turn, have helped to inform the wider analysis. As such, our experience of illness has given us a particular space and location within which to undertake this work that is not available to most people – therefore we assume what might be referred to as a true insider perspective, one that has accorded a degree of authenticity that hopefully infuses the work, while also being profoundly shaped by it.

## Autoimmunity

The immune system and its many irregularities has been the site of considerable intellectual interest, contest and challenge, although the history of autoimmune disease is surprisingly short. The earliest records of discovery in the field of immunology related to the fight against infectious disease and, while the human body was clearly capable of mounting immune responses to natural assault, it was not thought possible that the body would, in effect, turn against itself. The immune system was, therefore, perceived to be entirely benign. This notion was so entrenched that, for the first half of the twentieth century, the idea that the immune system could actually *cause* disease was entirely dismissed (Silverstein, 2014).

In a clinical context, the defining feature of an autoimmune condition is the manner in which the body perceives normal tissue as pathogenic. Ordinarily the human body is built to withstand invasions from foreign organisms (such as viruses, bacteria and parasites). Occasionally, however, this system can go awry; the resulting misdirected immune response being referred to as 'autoimmunity'. Describing the autoimmune condition rheumatoid arthritis, Felstiner (2007: 8) captures the essence (and essential paradox) of autoimmunity, stating 'it keeps treating body parts as aliens, keeps rousing immune cells until they are attacking familiars as suspects, picking on bones they are supposed to be keeping safe'. So, in autoimmune disease, the body produces an immune response to itself. In a world in which science has so successfully enabled our bodies to resist 'outsiders', be they viruses or bacteria, the notion of autoimmunity is utterly counterintuitive, yet conceptually most alluring.

In addressing the challenges (both conceptual and experiential) autoimmunity presents us with, we explicate and develop a number of overarching themes that articulate and interact with each other throughout the book: resistance and accommodation to autoimmunity; the existence of the pathogenic self; uncertainty and contemporary illness; and, finally, professional responses. The first of these themes, resistance, is reflected, first, and perhaps most profoundly, in the irony of a body that can so successfully resist the outside world (indeed, is medically and physiologically compelled to do so), yet is fundamentally unable to recognise itself as benign. Second, many autoimmune conditions are themselves resistant to identification and diagnosis. This is due, we would suggest, both to the shifting nature of symptoms and the systemic nature of the disease, which means that people are often engaged in something of a diagnostic lottery. In the context of living with autoimmunity, people resist and accommodate illness and its effects in a range of ways. Indeed, the everyday experience of living with illness is characterised by active resistance, struggle, accommodation and loss. Finally, as we will argue, the social work profession actively resists an engagement with the autoimmune body and its physical, psychological and material vulnerabilities.

The scope of autoimmune conditions is vast and 10 per cent of the adult population are affected by them, causing chronic, long-term morbidity and incapacity (Department of Health, 2012). There are in excess of 100 autoimmune conditions ranging from the familiar to the obscure. They can be divided into the more common conditions including rheumatoid arthritis, multiple sclerosis, type 1 diabetes and thyroid disease, and many more rare diseases.[2] They also include multisystem conditions such as systemic lupus erythematosus (lupus); endocrine diseases such as thyroid disease; diseases of the intestinal, hepatic and pancreatic systems; cutaneous diseases; and urogenital conditions. Rare autoimmune diseases are less well-known and many of the challenges in diagnosing, commissioning services and delivering care for patients are driven by the fact that these diseases affect small population numbers as individual conditions (Department of Health, 2012).[3] As with lupus, the gender profile of these other autoimmune conditions is predominantly female – connective tissue diseases 'all stick it harder to women' (Felstiner, 2007: 103). Indeed, a feminist analysis of rheumatoid arthritis (Felstiner, 2007) and lupus (Miles, 2013) indicate that gender fundamentally shapes the ways in which one experiences, lives and struggles with an autoimmune condition. While gender is, in many ways, inevitably infused throughout the autoimmune experience, it was, however, only one of many social identities that very clearly shaped our own respondents' narratives and experiences of living with the day-to-day realities of autoimmunity in a contemporary context.

The fact that autoimmune conditions affect so many people, yet are little-known or understood outside of the clinical specialisms in which they occur, constitute one of the central ironies of autoimmunity – they are simultaneously ubiquitous yet remarkably rare.

One of the effects of this phenomenon is that these conditions (like many other examples of women's health) attract little by way of health policy priority and research funding. A situation perhaps compounded by their traditional clinical location in the broad specialism of rheumatology. This irony is further reflected in the sociological and anthropological literature on chronic illness more generally, 'it is remarkable how often sociologists use autoimmune conditions to examine the effects of chronic illness even if the mode of pathogenesis is not relevant to their analysis' (Anderson and Mackay, 2014). In this book we seek to place autoimmunity at the centre of the chronic illness experience not least because it is through exploring the specificities of autoimmunity that we are able to understand and address the impact of what Cohen (2004: 7) refers to as the 'vital' autoimmune paradox. This second overarching theme lies at the very heart of the autoimmune experience. In short, the paradox focuses on the ways in which ourselves are both simultaneously constituted and undermined by autoimmunity. As such, it is those 'selves' that constitute the pathogen that threatens that very sense of self. That is, in autoimmunity, the self actively rejects itself – a situation constituting the most profound and intimate threat to our existential sense of security. The everyday consequences of this paradox (the existence of the pathogenic self), on living with an autoimmune condition cannot be understated.

One of the defining features of autoimmune conditions is that they are often characterised by symptomatic uncertainty and ambiguity and their impacts can draw in and out of focus as symptoms wax and wane. They are, by definition, clinically ambiguous (Napier, 2003) and are often difficult to diagnose (lupus, for example, takes an average of seven years) and some continue to be classed as 'contested' conditions – they are sometimes not fully accepted by clinical medicine as bona fide diseases (such as myalgic encephalopathy). As such, the range of autoimmune conditions can constitute enigmatic illness experiences for both patients and practitioners.

The uncertainty that these conditions generate and reflect is another core theme of the book. It is manifested throughout the experience of living with autoimmunity and is not only evident in the diagnosis, treatment and prognosis of illness, but also in its social, interpersonal, familial, public and private possibilities. The resulting constellation of biological and social effects are what might be deemed (and experienced as) vertiginous. The uncertainty and fluidity demonstrated by some autoimmune conditions very much reflects our contemporary social context in which the boundaries between health and illness are increasingly diffuse and difficult to determine and where illness and disease are a seemingly a permanent adjunct to 'health' (Bauman, 2000). Moreover, contemporary medicine has, at its heart, a determination to instil certainty and order onto uncertain situations and conditions. Yet, as Stockl

(2007) suggests, the drive for certainty only creates further epistemological disorder. We would suggest, therefore, that autoimmune conditions might usefully be understood as diseases of late modernity and that this contemporary context provides an additional exploratory lens through which to understand the contemporary lived experience of illness.

In addition to the personal and academic imperatives to explore the experience of autoimmunity, as social workers, we have been impelled to pose a number of questions to our profession's perspective on these issues. We have asked what place physical ill health and chronicity occupies in social work theory and practice. This line of enquiry has led us to also question the space occupied, in the professional consciousness, by the physical and social body. Perhaps unsurprisingly, we suggest that the answer to both these questions is that the space occupied by both the body and the everyday lived experience of illness without cure is negligible and configured in very particular ways. As a discipline, and a profession, social work is engaged in the process of change; change that makes a difference in both social and individual contexts. In the context of chronic illness, however, we would argue that physical ill health (lifelong illness) is all but invisible within social work's professional consciousness and, by definition, therefore, the profession is similarly unnoticed within the experience, and practice, of illness. While adult social work, in particular, deals very much in the frailties of the older 'vulnerable' body, commissioning and distributing resources, particular those that negate a person's need for long-term, state-organised service provision, it is remarkably silent on other critical indicators of vulnerability that may be the result of illness at any point in the life-course. Indeed, social work intervention more broadly is increasingly focused on intervention at either end of the life-course, being most visible in the context of child protection and adult safeguarding. Given that autoimmunity is apt to make itself apparent in the middle (and most productive) years, these conditions effectively bypass the policy imperatives that drive social work to focus almost exclusively on only certain forms and expressions of vulnerability. While one of our central aims in this book is to make autoimmunity visible, so too do we seek to assert the place of social work within that broader frame. There are, of course, many ways of operationalising the notion of 'social work' in both conception and practice (in thought and deed), and we, of course, recognise that the absence to which we refer is not necessarily entirely endemic.[4] However, our underpinning argument here remains; that the organising principles of our profession fail, to its detriment, to take cognisance of the realities of the physically ill body and, in the context of our discussion here, of autoimmunity in particular. In essence, then, in this book, the personal, the professional and the disciplinary coalesce, creating opportunities for an enquiry that will generate a space to explore and ask new questions of the everyday lived experience of autoimmunity.

## The semantics of illness

Throughout this text, we use the terms 'chronic illness', 'long-term conditions', 'lifelong illness' and 'chronicity' interchangeably, while remaining aware of the various meanings and debates embedded in these various terms. Manderson and Smith-

Morris (2010), for example, suggest using the term 'lifelong illness', instead of 'chronic illness', as a means of moving away from the previously dichotomous bio-medical categories of acute and chronic illness. Miles (2013: 7) states that this argument encourages 'understandings of self, body, and illness; and the struggles of daily life into a coherent "continuum"'. In the UK, at the time of writing, the language of policy is that of 'long-term conditions'; a turn of semantic vogue which we would suggest, has been unproblematically embraced, generating, in the process, a conceptual shift that has, arguably, sought to 'rebrand' the negative aspects of living with an incurable condition as personal challenges to be resisted, fought and overcome. This is reflected in, and by, both health research (which has moved from an explicit focus on burden, loss and deficit to living positively with illness) and healthcare policy, which now focuses very explicitly on the ways in which people should self-manage their health and illness. We would argue that this new language, ironically, does not, necessarily, foreground the experience of people living with illness without cure. Rather, it potentially undermines and obfuscates the very realities of daily living with illness that both research and policy seek to ameliorate. The language of 'long-term conditions' is not, therefore, our automatic language of choice, because the lived experience of autoimmune conditions explicated here is, without doubt, chronic, lifelong, long-term, without cure, ongoing and permanent. It is all these things and more. In addition, we refer, at different times, and in different contexts, to 'patients', 'service users', advocates', 'campaigners', 'consumers', etc. In doing so, we are neither medicalising nor diminishing the weight that can be attached to these terms and the assumptions and power that the purposeful use of language can generate (McLaughlin, 2009). Rather, we wish to reflect the nature of the relationships in the different contexts within which people living with autoimmune conditions find themselves – *people*, then, are variously 'patients', 'service users', advocates', 'campaigners', 'consumers', etc.

The chapters that follow highlight the four principal themes that have emerged from our analysis of our research data and the broader contexts of autoimmunity and professional practice within which we situate our project. Each chapter introduces a range of theoretical ideas, employing our data as illustration of the chapter's core themes. What we have done is to embrace an opportunity to bring together a diverse, and sometimes competing, range of literatures and disciplines into conversations that do not often occur in both academic and applied contexts. As such, while the experience of autoimmunity provides the central framework for our discussion, in the book, as a whole, we do not seek to provide an overarching metanarrative.

In the first chapter, we chart the history of autoimmunity and the biomedical and philosophical perspectives that underpin the concept. We explore the paradoxical nature of autoimmunity, wherein the self, rather than acting to protect it 'self' from disease, creates the physical and existential conditions for illness. This notion – the pathogenic self – is particularly telling in a contemporary context in which the boundaries constituting health and illness are increasingly difficult to determine. We go on to review the broader sociological literature on chronic illness in order to understand the place of autoimmunity within it.

In the second chapter, we explore the complexity inherent in acquiring a diagnosis of an autoimmune condition, which is often characterised by a lengthy period between the onset of symptoms and a definitive diagnosis. During this time, people are often required to battle to find a name for their condition, which, while perhaps uncertain, accords, at the very least, a legitimate illness identity. Here we employ our data to demonstrate the challenges autoimmune conditions can present to both patients and practitioners and suggest that, rather than being centred around a 'diagnostic moment' (Jutel, 2011), a diagnosis of lupus constitutes a process or a diagnostic journey characterised by uncertainty and what we term 'diagnostic vertigo'. This second chapter explores the meaning and impact of diagnosis for people living with autoimmune conditions.

In the following three chapters, we explore the experience of living with lupus, starting with the ways in which relationships with clinicians and other professionals impact upon the day-to-day realities of living with incurable illness. Here, relationships are played out in particular policy contexts (in the UK at least) and, in the third chapter, we chart some of the policy developments that have shaped the nature and extent of the clinical encounter. We argue that one of the, perhaps unintended, outcomes of these developments is the emergence of what might be termed 'patchwork patients' (Mol, 2002) and processes. Chapter 4, meanwhile, focuses almost exclusively on the data from our lupus project. In this, and the following chapter, our respondents' voices are foregrounded in order to help illustrate the ways in which people make sense of their illness and its day-to-day impact. We focus on the daily disruptions autoimmune conditions may generate and the ways in which people are required to manage and negotiate their day-to-day lives. We explore and illustrate the coping strategies people living with long-term conditions employ in order to manage pain and disability. This can be a particular challenge in autoimmune conditions, where the fluid and changing nature of symptoms demand continual vigilance and micromanagement. We are interested to understand the ways in which autoimmunity can generate simultaneous destruction and possibility and variously impact upon the everyday, taken for granted, aspects of daily life. We also further our analysis to explore the ways in which autoimmunity informs and shapes a sense of self. That is, the strategies people employ to attempt to reinstate the 'conditions of self tolerance' (Anderson and Mackay, 2014) and how they reimagine their biographies in this context.

The online environment provides an important setting within which to engage in biographical work, both individually and collectively. In Chapter 6, we explore the multiple sources and networks of support that play a pivotal role in the lives of people with autoimmune conditions. We argue that many long-term conditions have become digitally mediated illnesses and we examine, in particular, the support offered by contemporary technologies, as some autoimmune conditions, such as lupus (and other rare autoimmune conditions), are characterised by large, global, online patient communities.

Autoimmune conditions can have a profound effect on relationships and the family and in Chapter 7 we focus on the effects of autoimmune disease and the resulting changing roles and responsibilities within families and intimate relationships. Our primary focus for this chapter is an often neglected context within which the experience of chronic illness has been framed. We examine the ways in which the notion of 'family' has been considered in the health (policy and practice) literature and take issue with the ways in which the family has been simultaneously presumed and neglected in healthcare policy and practice (in a biomedical context in particular). We suggest that while the contemporary focus on patient management and self-care is underpinned by patient-expertise, partnership with practitioners, independence and empowerment, it ironically falls short of embracing the 'social' – that is, that 'family' remains largely absent. Further, we suggest that family relationships have been inadvertently marginalised, either through the application of the biomedical model or, ironically, through the invocation of the concept of 'carer' and we assert the need for a reading of the family that sits more centrally in our understanding of living with and displaying (Finch, 2007) chronic conditions.

The final chapter asserts the importance and role of chronic illness and the physical body in social work practice. We highlight the contradictory place of the body in social work where, despite its centrality to everyday practice (its management, control and organisation), it has never been more absent from day-to-day intervention. It is the chronic nature of autoimmune conditions and the very particular vulnerabilities of the autoimmune body that are invisible to the social work profession but should, we would argue, be central to its understandings of health, illness and vulnerability across the life-course. Here, most particularly, we argue for a reinstatement and re-centring of the body and 'body work' (Twigg, 2006) into both the theory and practice of social work.

While we conclude our book with a particular focus on the applied perspective and suggest ways in which the social work profession might more profitably engage with the issues we have highlighted throughout the text, this is not a handbook for practice. Rather, as we stated earlier, this text provides a starting point for both theoretical and applied interdisciplinary conversations about the complexities, ironies and existential conundrums presented by the notion and experience of autoimmunity. It is, after all, the experience of being chronically ill that sits most firmly at the core of the autoimmune experience and the central feature of the book is actually the exploration of what it means, and how it feels, to be a member of the 'kingdom of the sick' (Sontag, 2001). It is living with ongoing sickness, the day-to-day grind of illness that, while clearly socially mediated, is situated most forcefully at the foreground of people's experience. If the reader puts down the book having some new sense of what it feels like to experience a body so fundamentally at odds with itself, then our primary purpose will have been achieved.

## Notes

1 For a full account of the study see the Appendix.
2 Current figures suggest that approximately 400,000 people in the UK are diagnosed with rheumatoid arthritis (Arthritis Research UK) and 100,000 with MS (MS Society).
3 A rare disease is defined by the European Commission on Public Health as life-threatening or chronically debilitating diseases affecting less than five in 10,000 people. Rare single

autoimmune diseases affect approximately 100,000 and multisystem autoimmune diseases affect 50,000 in the UK (Department of Health, 2012).
4  We are referring here, in particular, to the practice of palliative care social work in which the visibility and ubiquity of corporeal dysfunction is both urgent and unavoidable.

# References

Anderson, W. and Mackay, I. R. (2014) *Intolerant Bodies: A Short History of Autoimmunity*. Baltimore: John Hopkins University Press.

Andrews, A. (2011) *Autoimmunity: Deconstructing Fictions of Illness and the Terrible Future to Come*. Doctoral thesis, Goldsmiths, University of London, http://research.gold.ac.uk/6920.

Bauman, Z. (2000) *Liquid Modernity*. Cambridge: Polity Press.

Cohen, E. (2004) 'Myself as Another: On Autoimmunity and "Other" Paradoxes'. *Journal of Medical Ethics: Medical Humanities* 30: 7–11.

Department of Health (2012) *Long Term Conditions Compendium of Information*. www.gov.uk/government/uploads/system/uploads/attachment_data/file/216528/dh_134486.pdf (accessed 9 April 2015).

Felstiner, M. (2007) *Out of Joint: A Private and Public Story of Arthritis*. Lincoln: University of Nebraska Press.

Finch, J. (2007) 'Displaying Families'. *Sociology* 41: 65–81.

Jutel, A. (2011) *Putting a Name to It: Diagnosis in Contemporary Society*. Baltimore, MD: Johns Hopkins University Press.

Manderson, L. and Smith-Morris, C. (2010) *Chronic Conditions, Fluid States: Chronicity and the Anthropology of Illness*. New Brunswick: Rutgers University Press.

McLaughlin, H. (2009) 'What's in a Name: "Client", "Patient", "Customer", "Consumer", "Expert by Experience", "Service User" – What's Next?' *British Journal of Social Work* 39: 1101–1117.

Mendelson, C. (2003) 'Gentle Hugs: Internet Listservs as Sources of Support for Women with Lupus'. *Advances in Nursing Science* 26(4): 299–306.

Mendelson, C. (2006) 'Managing a Medically and Socially Complex Life: Women Living with Lupus'. *Qualitative Health Research* 16(7): 982–997.

Mendelson, C. (2009) 'Diagnosis: A Liminal State for Women Living With Lupus'. *Health Care for Women International* 30: 390–407.

Miles, A. (2013) *Living with Lupus: Women and Chronic Illness in Ecuador*. Austin: University of Texas Press.

Mol, A. (2002) *The Body Multiple: Ontology in Medical Practice*. Durham, NC, and London: Duke University Press.

Napier, D. (2003) *The Age of Immunology: Conceiving a Future in an Alienating World*. Chicago: University of Chicago Press.

Silverstein, A. M. (2014) 'Autoimmunity: A History of the Early Struggle for Recognition'. In, I. R. Mackay and N. R. Rose (eds), *The Autoimmune Diseases*, 5th edition. London: Elsevier Academic Press.

Sontag, S. (2001) *Illness as Metaphor and AIDS and its Metaphors*. London: Picador.

Stockl, A. (2007) 'Complex Syndromes, Ambivalent Diagnosis, and Existential Uncertainty: The Case of Systemic Lupus Erythematosus (SLE)'. *Social Science & Medicine* 65: 1549–1559.

Twigg, J. (2006) *The Body in Health and Social Care*. Basingstoke: Palgrave Macmillan.

# 1 'I am my own worst enemy'

## Autoimmunity: diseases of the 'self'

In our introduction, we stated that this book focuses on what happens when the human immune system goes awry and in this opening chapter we begin to chart the ways in which it works to cause, rather than defeat, illness and disease. We employ this understanding as a foundation from which to explore the wider personal, social and political issues that can arise from the seemingly innocuous work of T cells, B cells and antibodies. We draw, in particular, on the work of medical sociologists and anthropologists who have mapped and theorised the experience of living with illness for which there is no cure. We employ this body of work as a foundation on which to build a conceptually cohesive framework to understand the experience of autoimmunity that, we suggest, is a particular point (and a very particular experience) where our biological and social selves come inexorably together.

Autoimmune conditions demand that, as human beings, we carefully consider our place in the world and complex relationship to and with it because, as we will demonstrate, the world can be perceived as a dangerous and risky place filled with all manner of possible biological (and social) enemies that must be actively resisted. As we will argue, in the process of partitioning ourselves so effectively off from the biological realities of the world beyond the body, the body, so ardently defensive, looks inward for self-generated threats and enemies. The critical point here, and one of our central themes throughout this chapter, is the profound existential and ontological threat an autoimmune condition may pose, given that it is our very sense (and biological experience) of self that these conditions so profoundly undermine – the body is, to employ a much-used military analogue in the context of autoimmunity, at war with itself. That is to say that, in autoimmunity, the biological self is (and actively becomes) pathogenic. The experience of the respondents who took part in our study and others (see, for example, Anderson and Mackay, 2014b) suggest that, in the face of this threat, people work very hard to reconstitute and rebuild the personal and social selves that are the collateral damage of these conditions.

This chapter thus explores the notion of the rejection of 'self' and the various implications this may have for a person's biological and social experience – the 'vital paradox' (Cohen, 2004: 7) lived day-to-day by people who have autoimmune conditions.

## Autoimmunity and the contemporary disease experience

The human immune system is a complex network of cells, organs and tissues that combine to work to protect the body from 'invasion' from natural (and man-made) pathogens. It is an evolved mechanism for enabling the body to discriminate between self and non-self constituents (Górski et al., 2001). Indeed, this fundamental distinction and the focus on self/non-self and identity lies at the heart of the field of immunology. The way in which the immune system operates is based, largely, upon the identification of those entities that can undermine human health and well-being that occupy the spaces in and alongside us. These entities or 'invaders' are, ordinarily, bacteria, viruses, parasites or fungi that can cause infection and disease. The immune system works to keep out these foreign entities or, alternatively, once they enter the body, seeks them out to destroy them. The 'innate' immune system (common to all animals) is the first line of defence. The innate immune system works by greeting bacterial ingress with white blood cells containing cells known as macrophages, which actively seek out and destroy bacteria. In humans, the innate immune system is complemented by the rather more sophisticated 'adaptive' immune system, most probably generated as a response to viruses, which the innate immune system is less capable of managing. In short, the adaptive immune system generates certain types of cells that, having identified a foreign invader, 'tag' it for destruction. This is done by other, specially adapted, cells (T and B cells). The system has adapted to recognise and remember specific pathogens so that, should the body be repeatedly invaded, it is able to kill the uninvited pathogens before they are able to create disease.

The immune system is at once hugely sophisticated, yet remarkably fallible in that it is able to identify and destroy a large range of potential infection-causing agents yet, sometimes, when it identifies harmless pathogens, including a range of naturally occurring allergens (such a pollen or animal hair), that it perceives to be a threat, it can inappropriately unleash a response that is, at best, unpleasant and, at worst, life-threatening. Moreover, and particularly apposite in the context of this book, the human immune system can also, contrary to the belief in the first half of the twentieth century that it was entirely benign, turn on itself. In this context, instead of producing antibodies to 'invaders', the human immune system produces 'auto-antibodies', that is, antibodies to itself – it thus perceives human tissue to be pathogenic, mounting, in effect, an immune response to self.

> While normally acquired immunity is carefully regulated so that it is not induced against components of 'self', for various reasons, when this regulation is defective, an immune response against 'self' is mounted. This type of immune response is termed 'autoimmunity'.
>
> (Benjamini and Leskowitz, 1988, quoted in Napier, 2012: 123)

The various effects of this immune response to self, known collectively as autoimmune conditions, can affect any part of the human body and, accordingly, when this happens, the potential impacts are many and varied. A conservative estimate would suggest that 5–8 per cent of people living in developed countries (this estimate is based on North American figures) may be living with an autoimmune condition and there are more than 100 autoimmune diseases currently recognised. Some of these conditions demonstrate a high population prevalence, such as rheumatoid arthritis and Sjögren's syndrome, while others, such as lupus, multiple sclerosis and type 1 diabetes, demonstrate a high population mortality (Rose and Mackay, 2014).

Despite the depth of understanding evident in the medical literature as to the workings of both the innate and acquired human immune response, the aetiology of autoimmunity has proved elusive and difficult to determine. Genetics, the environment, personality type, life changes and disruption, and the extreme effects of stress have all been linked to autoimmunity but, to date, there is no definitive answer that would explain why the human body should respond to itself in this way. While the range of autoimmune conditions present themselves very differently (both symptomatically and experientially), there are a number of common factors, paradoxically, and principally, the unpredictability and fluidity of their symptomatology and the fact that they are, for the most part, chronic conditions that are not cured but are managed (sometimes successfully, sometimes not) for the remainder of a person's life. In many, if not all, autoimmune diseases, symptoms come and go, moving into and out of focus, sometimes on a daily basis. They are notoriously clinically ambiguous and are the archetypal mimics and shape-shifters of the medical world.

As such, the experience of having, diagnosing and treating these conditions is enigmatic, to say the least. Autoimmunity is, put simply, a failure of the body to tolerate itself and, with this in mind, in the following pages, we explore the implications of this for people who are patently and demonstrably at odds with 'themselves'. We are interested to understand what this apparent failure of tolerance means in physiological and, more intriguingly from our perspective, social, economic and psychological contexts.

As noted above, it is only in approximately the past 50 years that the human immune system and its various aberrations and complications has come in for sustained attention. The very existence of autoimmunity was effectively in doubt until the late 1960s (Silverstein, 2014). Previous to this, the human immune system was considered inviolate. That is, as we have noted above, that it was not thought possible to confuse 'self' with 'non-self' or 'other'. Indeed, it is this distinction, or lack of, that lies at the heart of autoimmune pathology. It was, in fact, during the 1960s that the notion of an immune 'system' first appeared, marking a critical conceptual shift in the ways in which immunity was understood. The body was now not only responsible for reactions to allergens and pathogens, but was seen to have the ability to mount 'a cellular defense in which complex responses protected an autonomous self' (Napier, 2012: 118). The underlying assumption being, therefore, that the immune system works to simply identify and eliminate foreign 'invaders'. The elimination of difference thus sat at the heart of these dominant assumptions (Napier, 2003).

This is not to say that the notion of autoimmunity had not been considered up until this point. The early years of the twentieth century saw a number of discoveries that centred on a human autoimmune response, such as the discovery of paroxysmal cold haemoglobinuria – a rare condition in which there is an abrupt onset of systemic symptoms following exposure to cold temperatures (Donath and Lansteiner, 1904, cited in Silverstein, 2014). Further, one of the first to suggest that the human body might mount a biological attack upon itself was Paul Ehrlich who, in the context of experimenting in the wider field of immunology, coined the notion of 'horror auto-toxicus', pointing out that the human organism 'possesses certain contrivances by means of which the immunity reaction, so easily produced (induced) by all kinds of cells, is prevented from acting against the organism's own elements and so giving rise to autotoxins … so that one might be justified in speaking of a "horror autotoxicus" of the organism' (quoted in Gallagher et al., 1995: 50). That is, the organism is so 'horrified' by the notion of attacking itself that it will simply not occur.

The concept of autoimmunity was, thus, given relatively short shrift by a medical profession unwilling to overthrow the received wisdom that perceived the human immune system to be inviolate. Silverstein (2014) suggests that one of the reasons for this reticence was not the fact that the existence of autoimmunity was necessarily in doubt, rather, that this understanding did not fit the prevailing medial paradigm and that to address the issue would have been to challenge some of medicine's critical underpinning premises

> acceptance of a fact in science depends less upon its truth than upon its acknow-ledgement by the leaders in the discipline.
>
> (Fleck, 1979, cited in Silverstein, 2014: 11)

The road to a more comprehensive understanding of the autoimmune response was long and slow but, by the middle of the twentieth century, a number of develop-ments in the field of immunology could no longer be ignored. Animal studies in immunology were suggesting a mammalian autoimmune response (particularly in the study of thyroid disease) and, as a result, research began to uncover the basis of what we now know to be autoimmunity. Frank Macfarlane Burnet was, perhaps, the first to provide a theoretical basis for the concept of autoimmunity (Burnet, 1959) and he and Ian Reay Mackay subsequently published the first monograph that focused solely on the notion (Mackay and Burnett, 1963). They noted that autoimmunity could pre-sent in one or many organs (i.e., it was a systemic problem), that genetic factors were commonly seen, that these conditions had a female predominance and often had a fluctuating course – their work effectively marked the beginning of the science of autoimmunity (Roberts-Thompson et al., 2012). In the context of our interest in the ways in which self and non-self are ineffectively delineated in autoimmune condi-tions, Burnet's work is of particular importance. He was one of the first to focus, in detail, on the reasons why the body might produce antibodies to itself. For Burnet, it was not the human body's ability to defend itself against external pathogens that excited his interest, but the more philosophical question of how and why the body becomes unable to discriminate between *self* and pathogen. Anderson and Mackay (2014a: 148) suggest that, for Burnet, 'recognition of self represented the fundamen-tal biological problem' and his interest in the philosophy of this biological conun-drum effectively centred the notion of autoimmunity in the field of immunology.

What autoimmune conditions do, then, is to violate 'the categorical imperative not only of immunology but of most Western epistemology: self is self and not-self is not-self and ne're the twain shall meet' (Cohen, 2004: 7). The body, in this context, is perceived to be a coherent container of 'self' that is abstracted from its wider eco-logical context, a context that is seemingly inherently dangerous and risky and one that impels us to vigorously and vigilantly maintain our regulatory biological systems and borders at all times. It is a world full of potential invaders. This perspective, however, presupposes that, as those same human beings, we are separate and distinct from the world in which we reside and upon which we so obviously depend. Cohen (2009: 26) asks 'How did we come to believe that as living beings, "the body" sepa-rates us from each other and from the world rather than connects us'. After Cohen (2004) we would also refer to the work of Varela (1991) who makes this point suc-cinctly when he describes

> the intriguing paradoxicality proper to an autonomous identity: the living system must distinguish itself from its environment, while at the same time maintaining its coupling; this linkage cannot be detached since it is against this very environ-ment from which the organism arises, comes forth.
>
> (Varela, 1991: 85)

The ways in which biology and philosophy so clearly marry in this context is, perhaps, one of the reasons why the notion of autoimmunity, referred to by Anderson and Mackay (2014a: 167) as 'the dark side of immunology', is so challenging to under-stand (and explain to others) and is a concept quite alien to our understanding of ourselves and our corporeal and social relationship with that self and the world in which it so symbiotically resides.[1] Matzinger (1994) provides a nuanced and ecologic-ally persuasive explanation (and rejection) of the self/non-self paradigm that, she suggests, might have obfuscated the reasons why autoimmunity occurs in humans. She suggests that, rather than perceiving the world as one that consists of self and other (non-self), it is more useful to think of the dangers inherent in the events that stress the body rather than external 'things' that might threaten it. Matzinger's body of work provided a critical challenge to the perceived wisdoms of immunology and, in so doing, offered a view of the human body and its biological agency that is intim-ately connected to, not removed from, the world in which it exists. Cohen (2004: 10) provides an elegant overview of what this means in practice. Matzinger, he states 'helps reimagine the organism as a concatenation of biochemical transformations of energy and matter localised in the space/time which we call a life, rather than as a permeable frontier that needs to be defended'. Matzinger's (1994) call to reconnect us to our environment is particularly apt (and poignant) in the context of late mod-ernity, wherein the boundaries delineating self, society and the world in which they exist are, arguably, increasingly diffuse and permeable. This permeability, of course, is not one that reflects an appreciation of the ecological context in which we live, and the symbiotic relationship we share with our environment. Rather, it is one based on a keen awareness of the dangers the world poses to our state of being. Our relation-ship with the world, therefore, is based on fear and risk, ambiguity, insecurity, indeci-sion and fragmentation (Bauman, 2000). We would suggest, then, that the nature and experience of autoimmune conditions are emblematic of Bauman's notion of 'liquid modernity', which underpins an understanding of illness predicated on physical and existential uncertainty and significant states of flux (although we would caution a literal transposition of this notion given, as we will argue later, that the power structures that underpin illness and professional responses to it are tenacious and very resistant to change. That is, while policy imperatives and the political will may impel change in the medical field, the resulting sense of fluidity is, perhaps, more viscous than we might imagine).

In a society in which there are endless possibilities and myriad ways in which the boundaries of health and disease are variously drawn, the distinctions between health and illness become blurred and difficult to distinguish. Illness and disease, rather than being something exceptional that is contracted or acquired, seems to have no appreciable linear narrative. That is, there is no beginning, middle or end to it. Rather 'it tends to be seen as a permanent accompaniment of health, its "other side" and an always present threat' (Bauman, 2000: 79). Autoimmune conditions are, themselves, emblematic of this. The physiological and social circumstances that may generate autoimmune responses are difficult to quantify and isolate and the experience of having an autoimmune disease is akin to existing on this shifting health/illness continuum, wherein on any given day, the person may feel relatively healthy, the next very ill. The boundaries of health and illness, the ways in which self and non-self permeate and are subsumed into everyday life are, therefore, mutable and, in autoimmune conditions, as the disease process unfolds, these various boundaries can become increasingly difficult to discern and negotiate. Bauman's (2000) articulation of the ways in which 'others' are variously accommodated and, more often, resisted in the context of late modernity is particularly apt in this context. In a discussion on the mores of civil society, he suggests that managing the threats posed by strangers (others) is fraught with uncertainty and doubt, best managed by ignoring their voice, even if it is not possible to deny their presence. Bauman employs the analogy of the immune system here to suggest that, as we attempt to inure ourselves against the difficulties and problems, the 'risk-fraught commerce, the mind-taxing communication, the nerve-breaking bargaining and the irritating compromises' (Bauman, 2000: 105) that strangers pose, we leave ourselves open to other 'diseases'. He suggests that, as a society, we might prefer immunisation against 'invaders' – 'getting rid of the company of strangers seems a more attractive, safer prospect than the most sophisticated expedients to neutralize their presence' (Bauman, 2000: 105), but this, of course, carries its own perils because 'tampering with the immune system is a risky business and may prove pathogenic in its own right' (Bauman, 2000: 105). Bauman's analogue might be extended in a more concrete manner in the context of our analysis here, as we would suggest that one of the reasons for the apparent proliferation of autoimmune diseases in the twenty-first century relates to the fact that, as medicine allows us to (indeed insists we), resist neutralise, fight off and overcome pathogenic (rather than, in Bauman's terms, social) invaders, we become increasingly less able to effectively tolerate our own selves – that is, while our immune systems have been medically and socially manipulated to successfully resist the outside world, there is little we can do to similarly assist it to tolerate what occurs inside the body, which, in the context of the autoimmune response, causes, rather than resists, illness – an irony fundamentally at odds with the biomedical project. It is, thus, the self that is perceived to be intolerable, a concept we refer to here (as many others have, elsewhere) as the pathogenic self. In other words, and to marry both Bauman's (2000) and Matzinger's (1994) theories, by biologically partitioning the body off from the outside world, we undermine the structures by which we are linked to it and, at our peril, ignore the ways in which our biological connectedness might serve to protect, rather than threaten, us. We have become so successful at resisting invaders, therefore, that we are able to effectively resist almost everything (including, ironically, ourselves). Our contemporary immune systems are not, therefore, necessarily defective, rather, they are hugely successful and far too determined to destroy that which is perceived to be a threat. In the early twenty-first century, as human beings, we constitute the most stealthy yet profound threat to ourselves and, arguably, diseases that have at their core the rejection of self, provide the greatest challenge to our sense of ontological and existential security. This, we would argue, lies at the very heart of the clinical and personal experience of autoimmunity. Cohen (2004: 8) refers to this as a 'vital paradox'.

> Based on the assumption that under normal circumstances 'the self' ought to coincide naturally with 'the body' – or that at the very least the self ought to inhabit the living location of the body more or less unproblematically – this scientific paradigm depicts autoimmune illness and a living contradiction.
>
> (Cohen, 2004: 8)

There is a further irony embedded in the personal and chemical responses to autoimmune conditions, as Anderson and Mackay (2014b) suggest, while clinicians attempt to rehabilitate the autoimmune self through *lessening the reactivity* to the self through the use of immune-suppressants, patients engage in biographical rehabilitation to try to *restore* their sense of self they feel is displaced by their autoimmune condition. It is indeed paradoxical that some of us can seemingly only comfortably live with ourselves when that self is clinically and pharmacologically suppressed. Here, of course, we are conflating self and disease, but we feel this is appropriate in a context where, as we have argued above, the self is proven to be actively pathogenic.

It is the various paradoxes outlined above that lead us to our exploration of theories of chronic illness more broadly. This is because much of the research that has focused on the experience of chronic illness has, in fact, often been focused on autoimmune conditions, while not being explicitly grounded in that context. Much of the work that seeks to understand experiences of chronic and long-term conditions does so through the lens of various and multiple theoretical perspectives. We are no exception, yet we do this with the recognition that the autoimmune experience provides a further dimension to this reading.

## Illness without end

Susan Sontag (2001) famously referred to the fact that, as human beings, we are obliged to hold dual citizenship in both the kingdom of the well and the sick, as everyone, at some point in their lives, will undoubtedly experience the variety of ways in which illness will impact upon their physical, psychological and social selves. For people with autoimmune conditions, it is questionable, of course, whether they are able to traverse between the kingdoms, being more permanent residents in the kingdom of the sick (while sometimes being able to effectively 'pass' as a member of that other world). Stoller (2004), in his anthropological memoir of living with cancer, provides a moving account of the, sometimes uneasy, transposition between these worlds. Referring to the experience of remission in cancer, he focuses on the necessity to carefully negotiate the spaces in, between and around illness. We quote Stoller here, at length, as we feel his work draws out, in eloquent detail, the experience of ongoing ill-health.

> When cancer patients enter the zone of remission, it is not unlike negotiating the doldrums. You are in a space between the comfortable assumptions of your old life and the uncomfortable uncertainties of your new life. You have long left the village of the healthy in which sickness is a temporary respite from good health. Once you enter the village of the sick, as I have suggested, you can never fully return to the village of the healthy. During chemotherapy, you reside deep within the village of the sick. The routine of treatments and side effects consumes your conscious thoughts and soaks up your time... When you reach remission... you have the energy to walk to the gate of your new village. From your vantage you see the open gate to the village of the healthy. In your state of 'respite', you can leave the domain of sickness and walk the short distance to the space of health. People there know you and greet you. Even so, you realise that you have changed. People talk to you and wish you well, but you quickly understand that your time in the village of the sick has set you apart. You desperately want to live again in the village of the healthy, but sadly understand that your place is elsewhere. In the village of the healthy, you are surrounded by friends and family, but often feel alone. In the village of the sick, a way station on your journey, you are surrounded by strangers, but are silently bonded to them. They know what you know.
>
> (Stoller, 2004: 183)

Stoller's work, here, focuses on the existential experience of ongoing illness, the impacts of which have been variously drawn, with the burden, difficulty and disadvantage illness imposes being a primary focus of interest across disciplinary fields. Narratives of chronic illness like Stoller's have been the focus of enquiry in medicine, sociology and anthropology for many years (Blaxter, 2009; Carel, 2008; Hyden, 1997; Lawton, 2003; Manderson and Smith-Morris, 2010; Miles, 2013; Nettleton, 2013). Work that focused specifically on medical and functional definitions and understandings of the cause and impact of chronic illness, however, laid the foundation for a more nuanced and person-centred approach that has seen the narratives and experiences of people living with chronic illness take centre stage in research that focuses more on the existential, social and cultural contexts of living with a disease without cure.

A person's entry into (and anticipated and hoped for exit from) the kingdom of the sick is a well-worn path that has itself been variously mapped and theorised; most famously by Parsons (1951). The sick role – familiar, if unwelcome to most – grants a range of socially sanctioned deviant behaviours and societal responses abrogating an individual from normal social roles and obligations for the duration of their illness. In return, the ill person should seek medical assistance in order to recover. Once recovered, society expects the ill person to resume their previous roles and responsibilities.

Parsons' (1951) model is now conceptually ageing in the context of arguably lifestyle-related illness (when it is, perhaps, a person's own behaviours that might contribute to their condition) and the fact that the majority of people do not readily accept the questionable benefits the sick role might confer (in Parsons' original conceptualisation at least) and carry on their everyday personal, working and social lives while they are ill, at least if and when they are able. Similarly, Parsons' model has been criticised for its focus on the passivity of the patient and its insistence on the notion of presumed recovery. Parsons' original conceptualisation of sick role behaviour, then, perhaps best fits the experience of acute illness, where the person may well recover and continue life as before. Moreover, as we have noted, the kingdom of the sick is a place populated, variously, in the context of autoimmune conditions at least, by a seemingly endless and ubiquitous population. As such, it is not unusual to be ill – we are all variously ill – it is 'wellness' that is uncommon and remarkable

Nonetheless, the legacy of Parsons' (1951) work remains telling and, for those who are not likely to 'recover' from illness in the strictly Parsonian sense, but will continue to experience ill-health for the rest of their lives, this legacy can be particularly significant, as will be demonstrated at various points throughout this book. Part of this legacy, perhaps, is the tendency for early work on the sociology of chronic illness to focus, almost exclusively, on the negative aspects of living with ill-health. The negative impacts and outcomes were, until relatively recently, the sole focus of academic interest in chronic illness and a great deal of this work has focused on the functional limitations, deficits, disadvantages, disruptions and detrimental outcomes experienced by people living with long-term health conditions. Moreover, it has been the causes and the problems presented by illness, such as high mortality rates, increased poverty and an inability to work, rather than people's responses to, and understanding of, illness that have rather dominated the research agenda (Bury, 1991).[2]

Parsons' theory may, however, retain currency in the study of chronic illness by virtue of the possibilities of exploring more fully the conceptually separate notions of deviance and adaptation to illness (Bury, 1982). Here, the work of Gerhardt (1989) is useful in helping to generate and delineate these distinctions. She outlined two approaches to understanding the experience of chronic illness. The first, a model predicated on the stigma and crises illness may generate and the inevitable (and largely irreversible) changes in social status this confers and, the second, a negotiation model, which focuses more explicitly on the shifting nature of the experience of chronic illness. The person, in this context, does not necessarily adopt a deviant identity (as per Parsons' model), but adapts to the rigours and challenges of living with ongoing ill-health. The effects these challenges have on people were explored by Charmaz (1983) who focused specifically on the notion of loss of self in chronic illness. This overarching and endemic loss relates to the specific effects of living with a chronic illness, the restrictions illness imposes on daily life, the isolation people living with chronic illness may experience, the lack of legitimacy inherent in an illness that does not positively resolve and the negative effects (burden) that illness can impose on others. In later work, Charmaz (1995) focused not only on loss, but also on the ways in which people adapt to (and subsequently may come to accept and assimilate) illness. We would argue that, for those with autoimmune conditions, there is less of an experience of losing oneself, more a sense that one's self is fundamentally distorted by the autoimmune response. This generates a very particular understanding of the nature of loss and the impacts of illness. Loss in this context, as we will demonstrate in the following chapters, is often referred to by our respondents as a functional deficit in addition to a more existential absence. This point serves to underpin Cohen's (2004) statement that autoimmunity gener-ates a most profound paradox in that there is an overactive, dominant biological self that exists alongside (and can actively generate) a dissassemblance of that same self. At the centre of these adaptive processes are, perhaps, the meanings people, and society more broadly, attach to the experience of illness – a process of negotiating 'the mundane features of daily life dictated by contemporary culture and material conditions' (Anderson and Bury, 1988: 10).

In the context of the sociology of health and illness, it was, perhaps, Bury's work with people living with rheumatoid arthritis that exemplified the shift to a more reflexive focus on the experience of chronic illness. In a seminal paper, focusing on the ways in which a person's life is disrupted by illness, Bury (1982) contended that chronic illness is best conceptualised as a very particular type of disruptive event in a person's life. This disruption is far reaching and endemic, affecting a person's body, mind, relationships, work life, sense of self and identity, at the same time delineating and challenging the boundaries of love, intimacy and reciprocity. Illness, in this con-text, generates, what Bury (1982) referred to as biographical disruption.

Bury (2001) was at the forefront of the conceptual and methodological shifts in the study of chronic illness that have shaped our contemporary understanding of what it is to live with ongoing ill-health, and, by foregrounding the biographical implications of living with illness, he developed a theoretical framework that sug-gested that chronic illness fundamentally disrupts a person's sense of self and their understanding of the social world. That is, the meanings they attach to both are profoundly shaped by their condition. In this context, chronic illness represents 'the kind of experience where the structures of everyday life and the forms of know-ledge which underpin them are disrupted' (Bury, 1982: 169). As such, daily life and the taken for granted decisions, thought processes and symbolic and pragmatic daily endeavours are all fundamentally altered by illness. People respond to this biograph-ical disruption in various ways, but their social, cognitive and material resources are all mobilised in order to manage, reverse or otherwise ameliorate it. Biography, in this context, may be organised around illness and, the 'assumptive world' of the ill person and their significant others can, as a result, be fundamentally compromised (Bury, 2011).

Bury (1982) focused, in particular, on the meanings people ascribe to their physical and psychological circumstances, the consequences of illness and the ways (the styles) in which people adapt to, accommodate and/or resist their altered health status. The various disruptions a diagnosis of chronic illness can generate can necessitate a rethinking of the person's biography and, as a result, impel them into what Bury (1982) terms a 'biographical 'shift' from their perceived life trajectory, where there are relatively predictable chronological steps, to one that is unpredictable and potentially physically and psychologically damaging. The ways in which chronic illness impacts upon people's normative expectations and the manner in which it can alter the life-course and create uncertain futures was also the focus of Bury's work. Bury (1982) contended that the experience of chronic illness, and the ways in which it can undermine the structures and patterns of everyday life and the forms of knowledge that underpin them, can generate insights into far wider personal and social structures, norms and behaviours.

While this body of work focused explicitly on the experience of chronic illness, as noted in the introduction to this chapter, what it did not necessarily reflect was the experience of becoming autoimmune – experiencing the distinctly existential phenomena of finding oneself biologically, and fundamentally, at odds with one's own corporeality. Anderson and Mackay (2014b) suggest that, historically, one of the reasons for this apparent lacunae in the literature has its genesis in the clinic, where practitioners who themselves, only latterly having come to understand these conditions as 'autoimmune' in nature, are failing to communicate this to patients who, while perceiving themselves to be chronically ill, are either not encouraged to think in this way, or are simply unaware that their illness is autoimmune in nature. In their history of autoimmunity, Anderson and Mackay (2014b) state that in the 1960s and 1970s (the scientific growth period of autoimmune clinical immunology):

> few ordinary people felt a pressing need to understand the concept of auto-immunity; and accordingly, few patients perceived their disease as autoimmune. On the whole, there seems to have been a poignant failure in the clinic to communicate new, and admittedly esoteric, biomedical concepts during this period, despite the public ambitions [of scientists].
>
> (Anderson and Mackay, 2014b)

They go on to assert that one of the possible reasons for this seeming clinical reticence is the fact that it is difficult enough to communicate to someone that they have a long-term and incurable condition, without further suggesting that the genesis of that condition is, in fact, that person's biological self. The clinician has, perhaps, a difficult enough task in managing the realities of the illness without the additional responsibility of managing the patient's profound sense of estrangement from themselves that diagnosis of an autoimmune condition would suggest.

Bury's (1982) work, which remains the forerunner in an upsurge of interest in the sociology of health and illness, and in the experience of chronic illness in particular, was perhaps a rejoinder to contemporaneous work that had effectively abstracted the body and the experience of disease from the sociology of illness. In short, the work of Bury and others provided a shift away from a biomedical model of illness, privileging the lived experience of illness. As such, this body of work sought to relocate the experience of chronic illness more firmly in the body in a bid to reclaim the embodied reality of pain and discomfort from the ubiquitous deconstruction of the postmodern project

> the commitment to desire and discourse, including the de-constructed, deessentialised self and the endless championing of difference, has something of a hollow ring to it in the context of pain and sickness, disability and death: existential events par excellence, which expose the 'matter' of bodies, the 'limits' of discourse and the 'organic moorings' of identity.
>
> (Williams, 2000: 47)

Williams (2000: 47) takes issue with the way in which disability theory, in particular, has overlooked the reality of physical illness, tending to 'write the body out of existence', thereby obfuscating the physical realities of chronic illness within the sociology of health and illness. As noted above, Bury's work, and the concept of biographical disruption in particular, succeeded in placing the physical body, and the realities of living with chronic illness and pain, more firmly in the centre of the theoretical and empirical stage, although the notion of becoming autoimmune – becoming effectively 'allergic to oneself – remained steadfastly in the wings. As we will argue in later chapters, this revitalised perspective (on chronic illness and its impacts) was not one that was bound to infiltrate the applied world of social work.

While Bury's (1982) work undoubtedly reinvigorated the sociology of health and illness, his notion of biographical disruption has not gone unchallenged and, since its publication, the theoretical foundations of his work have undergone further development and refinement. The concept of biographical disruption has been variously problematised and, while it is a critical reference point in understanding the personal and social impacts of ill-health, it simultaneously has been criticised for its relatively limited theoretical and empirical range. In the context of the discussion here, Simon Williams' (2000) work is of particular importance. While acknowledging that the notion of biographical disruption is critical in understanding the experience of chronic illness, he simultaneously deconstructed the concept, shifting the theoretical focus to the ways in which biographical disruption and ill-health are interconnected.

Williams' (2000) specific critique centred on a number of related issues – the ways in which biographical disruption is predicated on an adult-centred notion of illness, for example (i.e., illness that strikes during mid to late adulthood, causing maximum disruption to normative life expectations and trajectories). It is also a notion, he asserts, that is confined to privileged, rather than disadvantaged, members of society (who are more likely to perceive the onset of illness as merely their 'lot' in life; one to be borne stoically, if not cheerfully). For some people, therefore, what is a critical disruption for others may be simply the mechanics of daily life.

Biographical disruption, in other words, carries particular class and age related, as well as ethnic and gender dimensions, which remain, at present, under-played and under-researched.

(Williams, 2000: 50)

This is an apposite point in the context of autoimmunity. Lupus, in particular, is clearly clustered in particular gendered and socio-cultural contexts. The diagnosis of lupus is undoubtedly more common in the middle (and, perhaps, most productive) years, but it also is more common in women (as are all autoimmune conditions) and particular ethnic groups (Afro-Caribbean and Chinese people). These socio-cultural variables may, in fact, be one of the reasons lupus is less well known (in the United Kingdom and USA at least) than some of the other autoimmune conditions that may have a more even socio-cultural profile.

Moreover, many people are able to trace their experience (and, for some people, their diagnosis) of lupus back to childhood. In this context, normative life expectations are those that already include illness. For people for whom illness has been an ever-present factor in their lives, therefore, other frames of theoretical reference are required to adequately explore and explain their experience. In this context, Williams (2000) asserts that a literal reading of the notion of biographical disruption, with illness presented as a precursor to the 'shattering' of our taken-for-granted assumptions about our bodies, ourselves and the world in which we live' (Williams, 2000: 60) does not adequately take account of the ways in which illness may already be, or become, a central constituent of a person's biography. It is the meanings made of illness and the context in which it occurs that determine whether illness is disruptive or, alternatively, simply part and parcel of a life already defined and shaped by difficulty and hardship.

G. Williams' (1984) research with people living with rheumatoid arthritis would certainly bear out this point. Again, while taking the concept of biographical disruption as a critical starting point for his analysis, he troubles Bury's (1982) broad-brush 'disruption' overlay, giving attention to the meaning-making of individual respondents. While illness, he contends, is an undoubted 'rupture' in a person's relationship with the world, people's own understandings and rationalisations for, in particular, the aetiology of their autoimmune condition is of particular note. Williams (1984) explored the ways in which people reconstructed their biography to make sense of their illness, asserting that it is the ways in which people understand themselves in the context of their world that determine their response to, and understanding of, their illness. Williams offers an alternative theoretical reading of the experience of rheumatoid arthritis, suggesting that people engage in a process of narrative reconstruction in 'an attempt to reconstitute and repair ruptures between body, self, and world by linking-up and interpreting different aspects of biography in order to realign present and past and self with society'. He suggests that identifying the causes (as opposed to focusing primarily on the impacts) of illness creates 'important reference points in the interface between self and society' (Williams, 1984: 197–198). As we have already noted, of course, when this apparent rupture reflects a dislocation from a presumed unproblematic corporeality and one's own relationship with the embodied self, the ways in which one seeks to reconstruct a relationship with the world might be very particular.

Simon Williams (2000) has gone further to challenge the underlying presumption at the heart of the notion of biographical disruption, this being that chronic illness *creates* biographical disruption. Williams, by contrast, suggests that the process can work both ways. That, in fact, biographical disruption can cause illness. Williams refers to a number of respondents in his own work whose experience would bear this out. Again, this is an important issue in the genesis and understanding of conditions such as lupus, as stress, and its various physical and psychological consequences, and negative (or positive, but nonetheless stressful) life events, in particular, are widely believed to create the conditions whereby the human immune system is more likely to go awry (see, for example, Winsa et al., 1991). Indeed, many of the people in our lupus study pointed clearly to stressful life events as the precursor to the start of their illness. Others stated that the experience of stress was often the precursor to a 'flare' of disease activity (a flare being the term used by both practitioners and patients to indicate an exacerbation in symptoms). Negative biographical disruption, therefore, was often invoked as an explanatory device for the ways in which the autoimmune body responds.

Williams also takes issue with the notion of 'biography' itself. Again, problematising the linear trajectory model that is suggested by the notion of biographical disruption. He suggests that life, in late modernity, is a series of never-ending 'biographical appraisals, revisions and improvements' (Williams, 2000: 61), which have a tendency to generate their own, very particular, self-reflexive ailments and maladies (such as eating distress and panic-related disorders). Again, these conditions, 'pathologies of reflexive self-control', he suggests, tend to be the prerogative of the 'worried well' and the middle class (Williams, 2000: 61).

Studies following Bury (1982), then, have succeeded in refining and reinterpreting the notion of biographical disruption generating, in the process, a more nuanced picture of the experiences and management techniques of people living with chronic illness. Biographical abruption, for example, refers to a critical 'breaking off' point that, in the context of life-limiting conditions, such as motor neurone disease, reflects the ways in which normal life effectively ceases when a person receives the diagnosis (Locock et al., 2009). Locock et al. (2009) make further reference to the notion of 'biographical repair', whereby a person is compelled, by the nature of symptoms and the inevitable deterioration disease causes, to continuously reset their sense of what constitutes a 'normal' life. People in their study sought to make sense of the life they had left and restore some sense of control, meaning and identity in a diagnosis of terminal illness.

'Biographical reinforcement', by contrast, refers to the ways in which a person's biography is variously confirmed and underpinned. In the context of gay men diagnosed with AIDS, for example, the diagnosis underscores their social struggle as gay men. For people with haemophilia and HIV/AIDS the same diagnosis, differently, but in a similar vein, underscores their lifelong experience of illness and physical distress. Their condition, therefore, serves to confirm (reinforce) either their minority status as a gay man or as a person living with lifelong ill-health (Carricaburu and Pierret, 1995).

For older people who have chronic health problems, in particular, the concept of biographical disruption may be less useful to explain their experiences of, and responses to, symptoms and diagnosis. In a study exploring the experiences of older people living with stroke, the notions of biographical flow and continuity are more apposite concepts that explain the fact that problematic life experiences are not one-off events. For them, illness becomes merely another issue to be managed in a life that may have been defined by hardship and struggle (both physical and psychological).

As will be seen later in this book, we would further translate the notion of biographical disruption to mirror the work of Faircloth et al. (2004: 245) who, in the context of stroke survivors in the USA, suggest that chronic illness (particularly that which comes on quickly, such a stroke) is better conceptualised as 'an enduring chronic illness narrative' that is 'part and parcel of biography'. Kelly and Field (1996) and Denny and Earle (2009) suggest that these developments and refinements on a critical theme best reflect profound shifts in society and the postmodern era that, as outlined above, is notable for its instability, fragmentation and diversity. The insecurity and personal and social ambiguity that are redolent of life in late modernity are further translated into everyday life for people living with autoimmune conditions, where uncertainty, ambiguity, doubt about the nature and extent of disease (and, for some, its very existence) are daily accompaniments to the challenges of managing what can be life-changing (and life-threatening) conditions.

These issues are nowhere more evident than in the case of medically unexplained, or, perhaps, more properly termed 'emergent illnesses' (Dumit, 2006) that are contested empirically, socially and psychologically. These conditions, perhaps most famously, myalgic encephalopathy (ME), otherwise known as chronic fatigue syndrome, and fibromyalgia, lack the clinical signs and symptoms redolent of clinically observable disease and, as such, their status as illness and the legitimacy this infers is questioned, their aetiologies are ambiguous and disputed; they are often perceived to be co-morbid; treatment regimens are unclear and their legal, medical, and cultural classifications are disputed (Swoboda, 2005). Researchers identify a number of these conditions as illnesses you have to fight to get (Dumit, 2006; Morris, 1998; Showalter, 1998). Unsurprisingly, they lack the legitimacy of medically accepted conditions and, for those people who experience them, they tend to generate great existential uncertainty.

As new conditions emerge in the context of both medical advance and political pressure, then, the need to further theorise chronic illness moves us on from Bury's (1982) conceptualisation of biographical disruption (essential though it still clearly remains). His original conception of the ways in which people make sense of chronic illness has been deconstructed to such a degree that the original conceptualisation is difficult to recognise or, indeed, reconcile in the context of twenty-first-century experiences of illness and healthcare. Discrete conditions and the variety of ways in which individuals manage their illness means that a blanket term is inevitably insufficient to provide a clear lens through which to appreciate and understand their experience. Indeed, in our study exploring the lives of people with lupus, we were able to identify many of the different facets of biographical disruption, appraisal, interruption, management and repair, etc., that are outlined above and, of course, the perpetual lived paradox that defines the experience of autoimmunity.

Taken at face value, the disruption caused by lupus (or, without diagnosis, its symptoms) is very clear to read in our respondents' accounts of the ways in which their illness impacts upon their everyday life, a common theme in many people's narratives was the fact that symptoms and the diagnosis of lupus created profound changes in their lives, creating 'sharp discontinuity in people's personal trajectories' (Lonardi, 2007:1621).

**Amanda:** Prior to diagnosis I held a senior nursing post but also had a 20-year history of fatigue, joint pains and what felt like viral illnesses. These would come and go, lasting for about three months at a time. As I had a busy life, I put these episodes down to overdoing it and being run-down.

As a critical care nurse, my concept of illness was very much set in 'acute, life-threatening conditions'. Hence, I didn't believe I was ill, pushed myself to keep on working and failed to ask for proper investigation into my health problems.

Three years prior to my diagnosis, these episodes increased in frequency and severity, causing me to have to reduce my working hours on several occasions. During this time, I was bullied by my ex-boss and officially disciplined over my sickness record. After having my third child I was simply too ill to return and chose to leave.

I eventually was seen in my GP's surgery by an ex-colleague of mine; who was shocked at the change in me and immediately referred me to rheumatology. The rheumatologist took 20 minutes to reach a diagnosis; telling me I had lupus and Sjögren's syndrome and these had been ongoing for about 15 years. The nurse in me fired off a load of questions and understood the diagnosis and treatment and quickly researched everything there was to know. Amanda the person was in shock and fell apart. During the next two years I put on eight stone due to steroids and immobility, could only walk 50 metres with a stick and needed help with everyday activities. My husband gave up work to look after me and we spent a very stressful six months sorting out benefits.

At that point I felt useless, worthless, a failure and could have really have done with some psychological help and support, but it just wasn't available. The adjustment from carer to patient was particularly painful as I was very fulfilled by my job. I totally withdrew from the world, not keeping in touch with friends or ex-colleagues. I was like this for about a year; until my husband and I decided that we would like something positive to come out of this and applied to go to university.

This was a real turning point for me in accepting my illness, as I felt I could achieve something; albeit a long slow process due to fatigue, pain and brain fog. I made new friends who had only known me ill and liked me for what I was. This was great at bringing me into the world again and I could see that everyone had some problems. It helped put my sickness in perspective and my peers often turned to me for advice. This made me realise I had valuable life experience, which I could use to help others.

In the last year my disease has stabilised somewhat and I am now in control of it. I have adapted my lifestyle and do not to push myself too hard or far; but listen to my body's needs. I eat a healthy diet, exercise gently, work within my limits depending on how I feel, meditate and go to bed early. I have lost four and a half stone and haven't needed my walking stick for a year. I also monitor my own bloods and am proactive about accessing medical help when I think I need it. I am back in touch with ex-colleagues and friends and I no longer grieve for my old profession.

Lupus is part of my life. It can be difficult, but it has taught me so many valuable lessons too. I like my lifestyle now; accept myself and would like to train as a counsellor.

Amanda's story exemplifies the notion of biographical disruption and to the questioning of taken for granted sense of self. The disruption to her body and mind are very clear to read in her account of her early illness, but her narrative also speaks of profound disruption to her sense of self and her particular place in the world. There are also critical indicators in her narrative that point to the disruption she experienced in her working life and her illness has forced her to renegotiate the rules and boundaries of everyday relationships – the shift from carer to 'cared for', for example, was, for her, a particularly difficult transition. In this process, the boundaries of intimacy, desire, sexuality and love were also tested and renegotiated. What Amanda's narrative also highlights is another critical aspect of biographical disruption; the ways in which illness and its effects are accommodated (or resisted) and subsumed into a new life trajectory that is, at once unanticipated, but is, nonetheless, embarked upon with new realisations and insights. Illness is undoubtedly disruptive, yet it is also incorporated and, for some people, subsumed, into a new 'normality'. For people with autoimmune conditions, however, this new normal may only be accessed or even glimpsed by effectively suppressing the biological self. It is, therefore, often necessary to supplement the person's own biographical rehabilitation with the clinicians' biographical work that, ironically, as we have already noted, involves suppressing the 'self' through the use of immunosuppressants. That is, the new self can only be generated when the old self is denied. The new normal is, therefore, a simultaneous suppression and restoration of self (the autoimmune paradox).

Amanda's experience clearly reflects and refracts many of the theoretical constructs we have referred to already in this chapter; disruption, abruption, repair and reconstitution. What we, through our very specific autoimmune lens, would add to this analysis of her account is a further theoretical notion, that of endogenous disruption, whereby it is the person's own self that, paradoxically, is both creator, resistor, rehabilitator and repairer of the various selves that experience the myriad biological destruction that autoimmunity generates. Amanda's body is in a corporeal state of flux, generated by her autoimmune response to her own tissues and cells. Despite this state of biological and existential disrepair, however, she comes to find a resolution of sorts in which her previous life is surrendered to the vagaries of her condition, yet, in the crossfire, she seems to have found a new sense of self and purpose. Amanda is, ironically, the destroyer, repressor and repairer of her biological and social self and, in the margins and spaces in and between these competing and contrasting states, she still manages to normalise, manage and subdue her condition sufficiently well to allow her to function and thrive in her newly drawn roles and responsibilities. Her sense of self is most certainly shifted but, perhaps, not ultimately lost. Our point here is that, in order to continue to live with one's self, it is perhaps necessary to try to reconcile the various selves that are at odds in autoimmune diseases. It is in this reconciliation that the normalisation of the ill self might be realised.

While Amanda's experience clearly illustrates many of the theoretical concepts we have outlined above, what her narrative also draws to our attention is the critical part played by the act of diagnosis in her illness trajectory. It is to this fundamental, if elusive, notion that we turn in the next chapter where we explore the experience of becoming ill, as the body, in often subtle, but nonetheless keenly felt, way begins the process of asserting its changing status on the lives of people affected by lupus and other autoimmune conditions. Becoming autoimmune and moving into and experiencing the kingdom of the sick, as we will demonstrate, is not simply a matter of identifying the nature of the malady and then responding to ameliorate its effects. Rather, it is a process undercut and saturated, like autoimmune conditions themselves, with ambiguity, uncertainty, fluidity, loss and change.

## Notes

1  For more on the history of autoimmunity, see Anderson and Mackay (2014a and b) Burnet, (1959); Rose and Mackay (2014)
2  The disability rights movement and the voices of patients, service users and carers have sought to challenge and provide a corrective to research that has traditionally taken deficits as a starting point.

## References

Anderson, R. and Bury, M. (eds) (1988) *Living with Chronic Illness*. London: Unwin Hyman.

Anderson, W. and Mackay, I. R. (2014a) 'Fashioning the Immunological Self: The Biological Individuality of F. Macfarlane Burnet'. *Journal of the History of Biology* 47: 147–175.

Anderson, W. and Mackay, I. R. (2014b) *Intolerant Bodies: A Short History of Autoimmunity*. Baltimore: John Hopkins University Press.

Bauman, Z. (2000) *Liquid Modernity*. Cambridge: Polity Press.

Blaxter, M. (2009) 'The Case of the Vanishing Patient? Image and Experience'. *Sociology of Health and Illness* 31(5): 762–778.

Burnet, F. M. (1959) *The Clonal Selection Theory of Acquired Immunity*. London: Cambridge University Press.

Bury, M. (1982) 'Chronic Illness as Biographical Disruption'. *Sociology of Health and Illness* 4: 167–182.

Bury, M. (1991) 'The Sociology of Chronic Illness: A Review of Research and Prospects'. *Sociology of Health and Illness* 13: 451–468.

Bury, M. (2001) 'Illness Narratives: Fact or Fiction?' *Sociology of Health and Illness* 23: 263–285.

Bury, M. (2011) 'Chronic Illness as Biographical Disruption'. *Tempus – Actas de Saúde Coletiva – Ciências Sociais em Saúde* 5(2): 41–55.

Carel, H. (2008) *Illness: The Art of Living.* Durham: Acumen Publishing Limited.

Carricaburu, D. and Pierret, J. (1995) 'From Biographical Disruption to Biographical Reinforcement: The Case of HIV-positive Men'. *Sociology of Health and Illness* 17(1): 65–88.

Charmaz, K. (1983) *Good Days Bad Days: The Self in Chronic Illness and Time.* New Brusnswick: Rutgers University Press.

Charmaz, K. (1995) 'The Body, Identity and Self: Adapting to Impairment'. *The Sociological Quarterly* 36(4): 657–680.

Cohen, E. (2004) 'Myself as Another: On Autoimmunity and "Other" Paradoxes'. *Journal of Medical Ethics: Medical Humanities* 30: 7–11.

Cohen, E. (2009) *A Body Worth Defending: Immunity, Biopolitics and the Apotheosis of the Modern Body.* Durham, NC: Duke University Press.

Denny, E. and Earle, S. (2009) *The Sociology of Long Term Conditions and Nursing Practice.* London: Palgrave Macmillan.

Dumit, J. (2006) 'Illnesses You Have to Fight to Get: Facts as Forces in Uncertain, Emergent Illnesses'. *Social Science & Medicine* 62(3): 577–590.

Faircloth, C., Boylstein, C., Rittman, M., Young, M. and Gubrium, J. (2004) 'Sudden Illness and Biographical Flow in Narrative of Stroke Recovery'. *Sociology of Health and Illness* 26(2): 242–261.

Gallagher, R. B., Gilder, J., Nossal, G. J. V. and Salvatore, G. (1995) *Immunology: The Making of a Modern Science.* London: Academic Press Limited.

Gerhardt, U. (1989) *Ideas about Illness: An Intellectual and Political History of Medical Sociology.* London: Macmillan.

Górski, A., Krotkiewski, H. and Zimecki, M. (eds) (2001) *Autoimmunity.* Dordrecht: Kluwer Academic Publishers.

Hyden, L. C. (1997) 'Illness and Narrative'. *Sociology of Health and Illness* 19(1): 48–69.

Kelly, M. P. and Field, D. (1996) 'Medical Sociology, Chronic Illness and the Body'. *Sociology of Health & Illness* 18(2) 241–257.

Lawton, J. (2003) 'Lay Experiences of Health and Illness: Past Research and Future Agendas'. *Sociology of Health & Illness* 25: 23–40.

Locock, L., Siebland, S. and Dumelow, C. (2009) 'Biographical Disruption, Abruption and Repair in the Context of Motor Neurone Disease'. *Sociology of Health & Illness* 31(7): 1043–1058.

Lonardi, C. (2007) 'The Passing Dilemma in Socially Invisible Diseases: Narratives on Chronic Headache'. *Social Science & Medicine* 65: 1619–1629.

Mackay, I. R. and Burnet, F. M. (1963) *Autoimmune Diseases.* Springfield, IL: Charles C. Thomas.

Mackay, I. R. and Rose, N. R. (eds) (2006) *The Autoimmune Diseases.* London: Elsevier Academic Press.

Manderson, L. and Smith-Morris, C. (2010) *Chronic Conditions, Fluid States: Chronicity and the Anthropology of Illness.* New Brunswick: Rutgers University Press.

Matzinger, P. (1994) 'Tolerance, Danger and the Extended Family'. *Annual Review of Immunology* 12: 991–1045.

Miles, A. (2013) *Living with Lupus: Women and Chronic Illness in Ecuador.* Austin: University of Texas Press.

Morris, D. (1998) *Illness and Culture in the Postmodern Age.* Berkeley: University of California Press.

Napier, D. (2003) *The Age of Immunology: Conceiving a Future in an Alienating World.* Chicago: University of Chicago Press.

Napier, D. A. (2012) 'Introduction'. *Cultural Anthropology* 27(1): 118–121.

Nettleton, S. (2013) *Sociology of Health and Illness,* 3rd edition. Cambridge: Polity Press.

Parsons, T. (1951) *The Social System*. New York: The Free Press.

Roberts-Thompson, P. J., Jackson, M. W. and Thomas, P. G. (2012) 'A Seminal Monograph: Mackay and Burnett's Autoimmune Diseases'. *The Medical Journal of Australia* 196(1): 74–76.

Rose, N. R. and Mackay, I. R. (2014) 'Prospectus: The Road to Autoimmune Disease'. In I. R. Mackay and N. R. Rose (eds), *The Autoimmune Diseases*, 5th edition. London: Elsevier Academic Press.

Showalter, E. (1998) *Hystories: Hysterical epidemics and Modern Culture*. New York: Columbia University Press.

Silverstein, A. M. (2014) 'Autoimmunity: A History of the Early Struggle for Recognition'. In, I. R. Mackay and N. R. Rose (eds), *The Autoimmune Diseases*, 5th edition. London: Elsevier Academic Press.

Sontag, S. (2001) *Illness as Metaphor and AIDS and its Metaphors*. London: Picador.

Stoller, P. (2004) *Stranger in the Village of the Sick: A Memoir of Cancer, Sorcery and Healing*. Boston: Beacon Press.

Swoboda, D. A. (2005) 'Embodiment and the Search for Illness Legitimacy among Women with Contested Illnesses', http://hdl.handle.net/2027/spo.ark5583.0019.004.

Varela, F. (1991) 'Organism: A Meshwork of Selfless Selves'. In A. Tauber (ed.), *Organism and the Origins of Self*. Boston: Kluwer Academic Publishers.

Williams, G. (1984) 'The Genesis of Chronic Illness: Narrative Re-construction.' *Sociology of Health and Illness* 6(2): 175–200.

Williams, S. J. (2000) 'Chronic Illness as Biographical Disruption or Biographical Disruption as Chronic Illness? Reflections on a Core Concept'. *Sociology of Health and Illness* 22(1): 40–67.

Winsa, B., Karlsson, A., Bergstrom, R., Adami, H. O., Gamstedt, A., Jansson, R., Adamson, U. and Dahlberg, P. A. (1991) 'Stressful Life Events and Graves' Disease'. *Lancet* 338(8781): 1475–1479.

# 2 Diagnostic vertigo

## Naming the illness experience

Clinical practice is underpinned by the process of diagnosis; it constitutes one of the foundations of modern medicine, being a central component of both its theory and practice (Brown, 1995; Goldstein Jutel and Dew, 2014). Diagnosis provides an explanatory lens through which to examine the experience, treatment and outcomes of illness. Moreover, it also serves an administrative and rationing purpose: determining access to service provision, insurance and restricted access medications (Jutel, 2011). The act of naming a condition thus operates as gatekeeper to a range of socially sanctioned, although questionable, benefits, not least the sick role and its potential for explanation, legitimacy and exemption (Parsons, 1951). The act and experience of diagnosis effectively demarcates what counts as disease from what does not and provides an explanatory structure in the midst of disarray. It therefore encompasses a range of functions and provides control for individuals by way of knowing 'what is wrong' (Jutel, 2011). For medical professionals, it is also a very visible function of power and control on multiple levels. It provides a way forward, dictating the type, amount and cost of care provision, it can determine the course of treatment and also, of course, a range of potential outcomes (Brown, 1995).

Diagnosis ordinarily exists at a very particular point in the illness experience, at 'a salient juncture between illness and disease, patient and doctor, complaint and explanation' (Jutel, 2009: 278). It follows that people who seek an explanation for their illness might anticipate a largely linear process (understood and anticipated by both sides in the clinical encounter), during which the person explains their symptoms to the physician, who then uses this explanation in conjunction with clinical observation and testing to uncover the disease at the heart of the experience. Jutel (2009) suggests that receiving a diagnosis is akin to having a road map in the middle of a forest – it indicates the way ahead, but not necessarily the way out. In short, it makes things clearer. What is difficult to understand is explained, management of the problem is suggested and assumptions can be made about the future. She refers to this point in the illness experience as the 'diagnostic moment', which is both 'transformative and contingent' (Jutel, 2009: 1). As noted above, there is a reasonable expectation that this 'moment' will be followed by other well-defined, socially sanctioned, moments encompassing suggestions for treatment and prognosis.

For many people with an autoimmune condition, however, this 'diagnostic moment', in which the type, course and outcome of their distress becomes clear, can be an enduring (and to be endured) process. In this context, the diagnostic 'moment' becomes less an easily identified point on the illness journey, rather, diagnosis becomes a journey in and of itself. For people with lupus, for example, the average time it takes to achieve a diagnosis is seven years (Lupus UK, 2012). For some people, of course, a prompt diagnosis denotes far more than the prospect of relief at knowing what is wrong and providing a route to social legitimacy. In autoimmune conditions such as scleroderma (a potentially fatal systemic disease in which skin, connective tissues and internal organs can harden due to the body's excessive production of collagen), and multiple sclerosis it may actually be life-saving, as the earlier appropriate interventions can start, the more likely the condition is to be successfully managed. The challenges autoimmune conditions, in particular, may pose for clinical diagnosis are well elucidated by Anderson and Mackay (2014):

> Modern medical diagnosis is predicated on disease specificity, the assumption that some singular disease entity is there to find. But the protean manifestations of autoimmune processes often defies any simply attribution of disease categories. When do diffuse aches and pains, a little morning stiffness, and a swollen finger become rheumatoid arthritis? At what point do intermittent tiredness, sore joints, and headache become systemic lupus erythematosus? What is the threshold at which muscle weakness, fleeting double vision, and loss of dexterity turns into multiple sclerosis? Occasionally a striking symptom might announce the disease. Transient blindness in one eye strongly suggests a diagnosis of multiple sclerosis; deformity of the fingers, rheumatoid arthritis; a butterfly rash across the face, lupus and recurrent jaundice, chronic active hepatitis. But diagnosis of the various autoimmune diseases is rarely an uncomplicated, quick exercise. Most of these conditions fluctuate in intensity, sometimes remitting, sometimes relapsing. Often they begin as a trivial problem, a mere nuisance, readily dismissed by those affected and their doctors. The illness can creep up on you. Even as symptoms continue, or recur, gaining significance in daily activities, it can be difficult to specify the disease. Frequently, the complaint seems vague and unfocused, withstanding efforts to fix it as a singular disease, rebuffing any diagnostic certainty.

The boundaries of what constitutes 'disease' are, of course, highly mobile and capricious and diagnosis is also socially and historically contingent, as Brown et al. (2009) suggest through their notion of 'social diagnosis' – a concept that connects illness both to social factors and social actors. A brief glance backwards in history provides ample evidence for this. Diagnoses of homosexuality, drapetomania and 'sluggish schizophrenia' are clearly historical artefacts, yet are testament to the ways in which medical diagnosis has been used to describe, and treat, 'conditions' that, with the benefit of historical distance, are clearly absurd. Weight charts and body mass indices (BMIs) are a further case in point, where small, seemingly arbitrary, shifts in the ways in which BMI is calculated and understood have the capacity to classify many more people in a population, for example, as obese. Diagnostic shifts of this nature have significant resource and policy implications for health services, not to mention the people who are 'newly labelled'. They also serve to illustrate the fact that medical conditions (diagnoses), are often presented as fact, but have, actually, 'a deeply grounded, socially negotiated genesis' (Jutel, 2011: 2). Highlighting the socially constructed nature of a particular diagnosis does not, of course, mean that the problems a condition causes do not exist, merely that it is necessary to be cognisant of the various ways in which an experience of physical or psychological discomfort or distress comes to be perceived as medical in nature. As Jutel (2011) notes, while the experience of illness may be very real, a diagnosis cannot exist until there is general agreement that the condition is visible, problematic and related to clinical medicine – all factors that are inextricably linked to social custom and belief.

This transformation is often governed by what a particular society, at a particular historical point, perceives as 'normal', bearable, anticipated or otherwise problematic. Similarly, diagnosis sorts out 'the real from the imagined, the valid from the feigned, the significant from the insignificant, the physical from the psychological' (Jutel, 2011: 4). Diagnostic classification is fundamentally a social act that has the potential to include and exclude. That is, conditions that are packaged into legitimate diagnoses can be confirmed with a measure of certainty, situating those on the outside as outliers, thus privileging some voices and not others, rare and contested conditions being a case in point (Jutel, 2011). Diagnosis is the medical and social sanctioning of the illness experience and, as noted above, is traditionally positioned in a very particular way, at a clearly identified point on the journey to illness and from person to patient.

Few of the respondents in our research project on lupus experienced a diagnostic moment. Rather, their experience of diagnosis constituted a journey that, for some people, had (and still has) no discernible end point. We suggest in this chapter that lupus, and many other autoimmune conditions, may unsettle and challenge traditional conceptions of diagnosis and that, in this context, the boundaries of power, knowledge and control in diagnosing and managing this, and other autoimmune conditions, are open to varying degrees of renegotiation and reformulation. We argue here that re-conceiving diagnosis as a journey requires that practitioners recast their practice of diagnosis to embrace the notion of symptomatic ambiguity and uncertainty, while they, and patients, radically shift their expectations of a 'diagnostic moment'. It is the nature of these diagnostic processes and the manner in which they occur, for people with lupus in particular, that are the primary focus of this chapter.

Here, we use lupus as an illustrative example to demonstrate some of the challenges which autoimmune conditions can present in the clinical encounter. We argue that the diagnosis of lupus is not a clinical event or a 'diagnostic moment'. Rather, it constitutes a process, a journey in and of itself, one that, for many of the respondents in our study of lupus, has no diagnostically satisfying conclusion. We suggest that uncertain diagnoses, such as lupus, illustrate the extent of the notions of both embodied and clinical doubt in autoimmune conditions and, concomitantly, throw into sharp relief the nature of the diagnostic process. This process, in the context of lupus, and in uncertain/contested conditions, such as chronic fatigue syndrome, fibromyalgia and medically unexplained symptoms generates, we would argue, a sense of diagnostic vertigo. Lupus, in particular, provides the perfect lens through which to explore the challenges, for both patients and practitioners, posed and addressed by contemporary clinical diagnosis.

## Systemic lupus erythematosus

As we briefly outlined in Chapter 1, lupus is one of a range of autoimmune conditions, wherein the immune system perceives normal tissue as pathogenic. The immune system becomes overactive and produces antibodies that have the potential to affect the normal working of organs and skin. It is a 'systemic' condition, meaning it has the potential to affect any part of the body. The symptoms of lupus, however, are not necessarily evident in every person with the condition and some people will have what is sometimes referred to as 'mild' lupus, while others will experience life-threatening symptoms and complications. The defining features of lupus are the widely varying range of symptoms and their fluid and shifting nature. Lupus has been termed 'the great mimic', in that it is often mistaken for other conditions. The range of symptoms, their sometimes transient nature and the variety of ways in which lupus can affect the body, means it is a condition uniquely characterised by symptomatic uncertainty, fluidity and continual flux and change. It is a condition that has the potential to create existential insecurity and uncertainty on both sides of the clinical encounter (Stockl, 2007), which, we would argue, is exacerbated by the challenges presented by the diagnostic process. The diagnosis of lupus mirrors the disease itself, being characterised, as we have suggested, by ambiguity, chaos, frustration and, for some people, iatrogenic distress; it is a process that, for the patient, may, in fact, constitute a secondary illness experience.[1]

Lupus renders orthodox and conventional understandings of the diagnostic process difficult, if not impossible. Diagnosis, as we have suggested, is not a clinical event (as it, perhaps, is more often in other conditions), but a journey that is often travelled slowly and that unfolds very gradually (sometimes over many years). The diagnostic process in this condition in particular is a complex interplay between the boundaries of knowledge/power, control, integrity and legitimacy which are continually (re)constructed and (re)negotiated between contemporary medicine, the patient and practitioner. As such, lupus poses a fundamental ontological challenge to modern medicine and effectively shifts and unsettles the ways in which we conceive of diagnosis – its social location and the meanings and potential outcomes inherent in the process. Indeed, the ambiguity and uncertainty lupus, and its associated idiosyncratic diagnostic process, reflects is the uncertainty and ambivalence of late modernity to which Bauman (2000), in particular, alludes. Shilling (2003: 3, cited in Nettleton, 2006) argues 'there is a paradox here: we live in an age when we have an "unprecedented degree of control over our bodies", but we are also living in an age which has thrown radical doubt about our knowledge of what bodies are and how we should control them'. Lupus is a condition that challenges the certainty for which contemporary medicine strives and throws into sharp relief the difficulties (for both patients and practitioners) associated with diagnosing, treating and managing conditions that have uncertain and contested aetiologies, treatment approaches and prognoses. Stockl (2007: 1550), in her own study of lupus, suggested that the ways in which modern medicine strives to create order 'generates more "epistemological disorder" instead of lessening it' and we would also argue that the range of autoimmune conditions, and lupus in particular, are representative of 'the epistemological changes that scientific biomedicine is undergoing' (Stockl, 2007: 1549). In this context, lupus highlights the dilemma between the scientific drive for clarity, precision and certainty and the ambiguous complexity of this and other autoimmune conditions (Mol, 2002). In the context of lupus, this diagnostic uncertainty and ambiguity has a range of pernicious impacts on the experiences, expectations and practices of both patients and practitioners, some of which we outline in this chapter.

While lupus is, to a degree, representative of a range of conditions that unsettle these epistemological changes, such as irritable bowel syndrome and chronic fatigue syndrome, it remains qualitatively different in that there exist, unlike these 'contested' conditions (which Dumit (2006: 578) refers to as 'biomental'), clear diagnostic criteria and biological markers that are said to be indicative of a diagnosis of lupus – such as the existence of certain auto antibodies in the blood (anti-nuclear antibodies, anti-DNA antibodies and a range of extractable nuclear antigens). As noted earlier, however, despite these clinical markers (which, it should be stressed, not all people experiencing/diagnosed with the condition exhibit at all times), the data from our study suggests that the diagnosis of lupus is characterised by the propensity for missed diagnosis and misdiagnosis.

Many of the people who we spoke to referred to the uncertainty they faced when seeking a diagnosis and our data demonstrate that, for people with lupus, there may be a critical disconnection between expectations of what the diagnostic process can achieve and their experience of it. Patients have a reasonable expectation that a consultation (or series of consultations) will uncover the clinical reason/s for their illness (Dumit, 2006; Jutel, 2009; Nettleton, 2006; Stockl, 2007). They would anticipate that medicine would 'know what to do' in the face of their distress. There will be a concomitant expectation that the patient will also 'know what to do' following diagnosis, for they will have an explanation (a diagnosis), a plan of action and a range of potential outcomes. Much of this knowledge is, traditionally, garnered from within the consultation itself, through and by the relationship with the practitioner. Roles and relationships in this context are predetermined and well-drawn with clear points of authority delineated – by taking a stance with a diagnosis, for example, the doctor is asserting his/her authority. Olson and Abeysinghe (2014: 51) suggest that doctors continue to be trained for certainty in an uncertain world. Fostering certainty, they argue, may be done to instil confidence, but 'it can lead clinicians to ignore contradictory evidence, [lack] sensitivity to variation and [be] intolerant of ambiguity'. When the diagnosis is not certain, or when there is no diagnosis or explanation forthcoming, the patient is often left to manage that uncertainty alone, sometimes taking on the role of the 'proto-professional', where, in the absence of clinical certainty, they are required to actively 'participate in the process of being diagnosed and cured' (Novas and Rose, 2000; Stockl, 2007:1557).

## The experience of diagnosis

The pervasive and intrusive effects of lupus were clearly evident in all our respondents' narratives. Symptoms varied from mild to life-threatening and included (to name only a small selection) an inability to move and speak coherently, multi-coloured rashes, chronic fatigue, joint pain, depression, weight loss, headache, widespread and unexplained pain, mouth ulcers, cognitive difficulties, paralysis, alopecia, pneumonia, infections, miscarriage (a common occurrence for women with lupus), pleurisy, kidney failure and heart attack.

The variety and range of symptoms people reported meant that lupus was often a diagnosis of exclusion – many people ran a gamut of possible diagnoses before lupus was offered as an explanation for their illness, which effectively permeated every aspect of everyday life. Charlotte and Amanda's stories exemplify the lupus maze of uncertainty, ambiguity and the battle for legitimacy they felt impelled to engage in.

> **Charlotte:** I couldn't move or speak coherently. I also had a rash all over my body which looked purply/red. They thought I had Guillain Barre syndrome, then a stroke, then MS… I was in hospital for three weeks. They even said maybe my problem was psychiatric…
>
> This did upset me as I felt it was all in my head and not real pain I was feeling. I did think I was going mad. I discharged myself and went home but needed social services to help with carers to come in and help with cooking, cleaning, etc., for nearly six months… it was awful…
>
> After this I just kept getting bronchitis, chest infection, pleurisy, viral infections etc. All the hospital said was take paracetamol and bed rest. I was then told I was having migrainous seizures. I was then referred to a rheumatologist who prescribed plaquenil due to my skin rashes in the sun and joint pains. They concluded that I had a lupus-like illness but were reluctant to fully diagnose this. I am now 38 years old and have had to leave full-time jobs at least three times due to this.

What Charlotte's story and the following excerpt from Amanda's also demonstrate is not only the pervasive yet elusive nature of the lupus, but also the enigmatic nature of its diagnosis. This, perhaps, reflects the fact that, despite the clinical markers that identify it as a bona fide autoimmune condition, people appear to experience pervasive difficulties in acquiring a diagnostic label

> **Amanda:** From the age of about 23, I would suffer from episodes of chronic fatigue, joint pain, depression and general malaise. I put these down to viral illness caused by stress, being run-down, etc., as I had a busy life. During my first marriage when these episodes occurred, my then-husband, would say I was, lazy, attention-seeking and a hypochondriac. After my divorce eight years ago, these episodes became more frequent and severe and, although at times blood tests showed high inflammatory markers, I was never tested for autoimmune specific bloods or referred to a rheumatologist. Hence I still attributed this to stress and being run-down. This was despite the fact that I needed maximum doses of

paracetamol and ibuprofen every day just to get through the working day and that the pain and fatigue would only really ease after a couple of glasses of wine in the evening.

I moved house a fair bit between five and eight years ago and with each GP I did mention my symptoms, which were concerning me at this stage. However the diagnoses varied from, ME, depression, viral illness, hypochondria and even alcoholism.

Olson and Abeysinghe (2014: 54) suggest that general practice is the speciality that most encounters uncertainty – patients are referred onwards to specialists for a more certain diagnosis. If, however, the uncertainty within general practice acts as barrier rather than a springboard to referral, patients can remain in 'diagnostic limbo' (Corbin and Strauss, 1985). Charlotte and Amanda's accounts also reflect their search to legitimise their undiagnosed illness and, when this is seemingly not possible, their physicians codified their illness as psychogenic in origin, a not uncommon experience.

Indeed, one of the ways in which clinicians appeared to overcome their own uncertainty (and, perhaps, a measure of the ways in which they took opportunities to reassert their power in the patient/practitioner relationship) was to turn to psychogenic explanations for people's experiences, when biological explanations were not forthcoming or were effectively discounted. In this context, practitioners sometimes found it difficult to shift their clinical gaze from the patient's mental health. Psychiatry, for many of our respondents, has provided a convenient, but often damaging, fallback position for clinicians uncertain as to the nature, extent and presentation of lupus symptoms. As a result, some people felt an obligation to have to 'prove' they were ill in an attempt to wrestle legitimacy from a situation that profoundly undermined both their experience and their integrity, sometimes resulting in what might be described as iatrogenic consultations. Rose's story demonstrates this phenomenon.

**Rose:** My symptoms started around six months after the birth of my second child, following a severe mastitis infection. The symptoms I had were that I was overwhelmingly tired, aching all over with pain that was widespread, I lost a lot of weight over a few months, I had headaches, mouth ulcers, difficulty concentrating, wasn't able to sleep and generally felt pretty rubbish. I visited my GP with these symptoms after they had persisted for around three months. My GP promptly (mis)diagnosed me with postnatal depression and sent me off with antidepressants. When my symptoms did not improve he sent me to a psychiatrist, who threatened to have me sectioned because I wasn't getting better quickly enough, oh, and when I said that I wasn't depressed he said that I was saying that because I was depressed! So, I pretended to be better, as the thought of being sectioned when I had a toddler and a baby didn't strike me as a good option.

I feel that being (mis)diagnosed with a mental illness for several years was damaging because (a) it meant that I wasn't getting medical treatment that would have improved my illness, I wonder if my lupus would be less severe if it had been treated correctly earlier; (b) being 'labelled' with a mental illness diagnosis was very hard, nobody listened to me, I was given drugs that didn't help, and when I wasn't getting better was threatened with a section and ECT treatment. I feel as though the diagnosis I was given stopped the medical profession from looking beyond that label, and interpreting all of my symptoms within the context of that diagnosis.

For Rose and other respondents, accounts of their condition were treated with caution; their own narratives and voices silenced and their understanding of their illness discounted and marginalised. Atkins (2010, cited in Olson and Abeysinghe, 2014: 51–52) describes a similar experience in relation to her autoimmune condition, myasthenia gravis, which remained undiagnosed for ten years – her paralysis was attributed to psychological rather than physical causes.

> Confronted by a difficult and ambiguous case, most doctors and nurses routinely grasped for certainty rather than attempting to tolerate any ambivalence. It was easier to categorise me as a 'head case' than to accept I was suffering from an atypical and life-threatening illness about which they had very limited understanding and control.

People interviewed in our study responded to the complexities of diagnosing lupus in a range of ways. Some accepted the various explanations that were forthcoming from practitioners; diagnoses that changed and shifted during and between consultations. Others actively resisted what they perceived to be an oppressive diagnostic process and, in doing so, embodied a contemporary patient role that is increasingly complex and multifaceted. The work of Mendelson (2006, 2009) and, more recently, Miles (2013) on women's experiences of living with lupus, points to the gendered dimension of acquiring a diagnosis. Mendelson (2009: 390) suggests that women face a long period of diagnosis as their symptoms are dismissed as 'somatic expressions of stress'. As one woman in her research commented, '[I was] mostly being diagnosed with Disaffected Housewife Syndrome, my name for what male doctors see as a women's [sic] problem of complaining of being sick when he believed they really weren't (often on first sight)'. Gender is an underpinning explanation for women's experiences of struggling to acquire a diagnosis but so too is the complexity of autoimmunity and the clinical encounter, itself shaped by gender power relations.

While the power within the diagnostic process lies, then, primarily on the professional side of the patient/practitioner relationship, there have been some contemporary changes in the ways in which medical knowledge and diagnostic power are distributed and enacted. Nettleton (2004) frames this metamorphosis in a number of broad sociological changes, most notably the shift towards widely available, web-based, information that allows the patient previously privileged information and knowledge and the concomitant power that this knowledge confers. Not only has medicine escaped the bounds of the hospital and other medical institutions, she notes, but the manner of its production has also changed immeasurably. Critical consumers of healthcare, rather than simply accessing medical information are also now the producers of medical knowledge.

As we discuss more fully in Chapter 6, the internet, for example, has opened up new and multiple ways of understanding and knowing that are readily accessible and easily navigated. Webpages addressing every possible autoimmune condition abound and there are multiple sources and networks of support that can play a pivotal role in the lives of those diagnosed and those seeking an explanation for their experiences of illness. The resulting internet communities have enabled patients to develop techniques for managing life with a chronic illness and, for some of our respondents, it was from online sources and communities that they garnered critical information about their condition and, for some, a more certain route to diagnosis.

The contemporary patient brings privileged experiential knowledge to the clinical encounter and the possibility of accessing a considerable amount of information long before it occurs. The power of the clinician shifts in this context and the patient arguably becomes a partner in clinical decision-making, 'the relationship is no longer a one-way power-dependency relationship but an encounter based on knowledge (albeit unequal) about health and disease' (Jutel, 2011: 69). But, as we argue in Chapters 3 and 6, clinicians and patients alike do not always welcome or embrace this shift. Some of our respondents' narratives highlight the power struggle at the base of this shift very clearly and, while some practitioners were willing to engage with patients within these newly delineated relationships, others actively resisted new forms of clinical encounter. Similarly, some patients assumed the role of 'proto-professional' easily, while others preferred to maintain a more traditional doctor/patient relationship.

A notable outcome of these contemporary means of accessing, using and producing medical information is the possibility of diagnosing oneself. For many of our respondents, however, this was not a proactive or affirming endeavour. Rather, it was a response to what people perceived to be incorrect or absent diagnoses, alongside insufficient evidence that their illness experience was validated by clinicians. Losing faith in traditional approaches to diagnosis, patients armed themselves with alternative sources of knowledge and engaged in a battle with their practitioners, determined to achieve a diagnosis (and treatment), or at least an explanation for their illness experience. The information respondents garnered from alternative sources led many to attend consultations replete with information about lupus, indeed some respondents referred to a process in which they felt it necessary to actively educate their GP about the condition. Still, it seems the legitimacy of their experience and the knowledge they had about their condition was challenged and consistently undermined.

Dana's story highlights these issues quite starkly and also demonstrates a further theme that was a common feature of respondents' experiences of diagnosis – the notion of diagnosis by hindsight.

> **Dana:** I guess I first experienced symptoms of lupus when I was away at university. The fatigue was probably the most prevalent symptom in those days, but being a student I put it down to lectures, working and partying... I couldn't cope with the tiredness and it resulted in my becoming depressed and dropping out.

Then, ten years later, the fatigue became something more. Infections became more common; mouth ulcers, bone and muscle pain – particularly joints, Reynaud's in my hands initially and then in my feet – at first mild then severe. Headaches, confusion, memory loss, fever in the night. Rashes started appearing.

Backwards and forwards to the doctors I went. You're depressed they would say. Why am I depressed was my reply. I have a lovely home, lovely job, lovely marriage. You're anaemic was the next one. Finally, after talking to my dad, I put two and two together. He has autoimmune problems, maybe I did too.

Six months later, I can't move for pain, even if I could I was too exhausted to want to move. My life was hell. Finally, a doctor referred me to the hospital. I think he just wanted to shut me up. More blood tests. First appointment with a registrar. Registrar says to me... I think you could have lupus. Hallelujah! I think. Off I trot for more tests. Go back one month later – different registrar – no you don't have lupus, you have fibromyalgia and all I will do is put you on antidepressants. He took one look at my notes that said I had had depression and made his mind up. Even when I got upset he just brushed me aside.

Six months later, I'm back at the doctors pleading for help. My employers were now getting shirty about me having time off, I felt friends and family had washed their hands of me and all through my pain and tiredness I had to keep going.

After much persuasion, Dana's GP offered an anti-nuclear antibody test and she was eventually diagnosed with lupus.

In the absence of a timely or satisfying clinical response to symptoms, self-diagnosis, using alternative sources of information or hindsight, was often a prerequisite to a more formal diagnostic process, but patients were required to battle, first to prove the existence of their illness and, second, to persuade those with the most power in the clinical encounter that their experience of illness was valid. While the changing boundaries of knowledge and power inextricably impact upon both practitioner and patient, and even as the patient assumes new roles and responsibilities within the clinical encounter, therefore, traditional hierarchies remain (Jutel, 2011). While medicine tolerates the newly informed consumer, it retains, for our respondents, the upper hand in the power play between users/consumers and purveyors of medicine. Many people reported the battle they felt they were engaged in as a damaging, iatrogenic experience in which not only their integrity but also their sense of self was challenged on multiple levels.

## Diagnosis and the illness identity

The diagnostic process serves to demarcate the personal and social movement from person to patienthood (Sayce, 1999), in which the ill person assumes a new 'illness identity' that may include unforeseen changes to their life expectations and the roles and relationships within it, becoming, in the process, a citizen in the 'kingdom of the sick' (Sontag, 2001: 3). A person's sense of self is, thus, variously realigned in the context of ill health, 'in a person suffering severe or chronic illness, just as in a community suffering an epidemic, disease provokes a crisis of self-definition; internal boundaries shift, and the complex structures of identity rearrange themselves' (Klinkenborg,

1994: 78, in Jutel, 2011). In addition, anticipated and expected life stages and events are reassessed in the context of ongoing ill-health, patients are thus required to find new meaning in the changing relationship between their familiar self and their developing identity as a person with an illness (Stockl, 2007). As Stoller (2004: 65) says: 'The process of diagnosis, of course, erases certainty from a person's life. The possibility of serious illness involuntarily throws you into a fast moving stream, the current of which is carrying you to an uncertain destination.'

Many respondents reflected upon the ways in which illness and the lupus diagnosis impacted upon their sense of self and the ways in which they accommodated and/or resisted an illness identity. Amanda clearly outlines these issues:

> The effect of lupus on my identity has been the most difficult and painful aspect to come to terms with. Prior to being diagnosed I held a senior nursing post and would have described myself as confident, independent, extrovert, hardworking and dynamic. I was good at my job, loved working in a caring, therapeutic role and derived a lot of self-esteem from my job.
>
> … Although I had symptoms for 15 years before I was diagnosed, they didn't affect my lifestyle until four years before I was diagnosed and three years before I had to leave nursing. During those three years, I had repeated episodes of sick leave. As I had no 'official diagnosis' but was off sick with non-specific symptoms, I was given no support at all by the organisation I worked for. My boss bullied me and harassed me at home while I was sick. When I returned to work I was disciplined over my 'appalling' sickness record.
>
> … Eventually I left that post as the stress of the bullying was making me more sick. I worked part-time on the nurse bank for the next three years, gradually reducing my hours until I couldn't even manage two four-hour shifts a week. Because I left of my own accord and had worked so few weekly hours the past two years, I was not entitled to incapacity benefit, income support or my occupational pension.
>
> When I was diagnosed with lupus, I realised I would never be able to return to nursing and on top of that the pain and immobility meant I couldn't do simple everyday tasks for myself or children.

Amanda's excerpt also indicates the ways in which diagnosis performs regulatory and gatekeeping functions; determining the legal basis for the provision of services and employment rights the person is permitted access to (Brown, 1995). At an individual level, diagnosis legitimises illness and forms the basis for the allocation of resources, from welfare support through access to treatment and pharmaceuticals (Jutel, 2011).

Diagnosis (or the absence thereof), therefore, functions to provide a structure to the redefinitions of self, identity and purpose that chronic illness can impose. It can provide a lens through which to examine what Brown (1995: 46) referred to as the 'rupture' that chronic disease can cause in a person's relationship with the world. A diagnostic label not only makes sense of symptoms, but also helps to frame a person's response to their experience of illness. Goldstein Jutel (2014: 82) states that, following diagnosis, a prognosis can be made that has a powerful impact on identity. Prognosis, she says, 'sets a blueprint for the future competing with, challenging, and shifting one's life story, personal values, and intentions. Future direction is modified, compromised or even non-existent.'

For people in our study without a formal diagnosis, or for whom there was no explanatory framework for their experience, the lack of a diagnosis often assumed an effective barrier to coming to terms with their condition. They were left in a most unsatisfying position, knowing that their illness was very real, while lacking a clinical frame of reference that might help make sense of their experience.

Some respondents took a very different approach to the labelling process, however, actively resisting a formal diagnosis and the ways in which it may impact upon their sense of self and everyday life. For some, therefore, diagnosis was to be challenged, rather than sought and/or embraced. Arguably, patients who move from one practitioner to another, and who seek alternative perspectives and repeated consultations are not just struggling to access a diagnosis but also potentially resisting one.

The power of a diagnostic label, whether one would seek or resist it, is very clear. This power makes the process of diagnosis 'an important site of contest and compromise', which confers power largely to the professional in the doctor/patient relationship (Jutel, 2011: 5). Diagnosis lies at the heart of this relationship and determines how individuals begin to make sense of their illness experience. Indeed, as Jutel (2011) notes, it is the process that actually brings the patient and the doctor relationship into being, the nature of that relationship being mediated by a range of sometimes unknowable variables where the patient and practitioner may actually be addressing the same problem from radically – and sometimes irrevocably – different perspectives.

What has become apparent is that diagnosis, for many of the respondents in our study, was not an 'event'. It did not constitute a recognisable 'moment' in their illness journey, as is the case with many other chronic and long-term conditions. Indeed, it is the diagnostic response to other conditions that shapes the expectations of an immediate and straightforward diagnostic event in others. For our respondents, diagnosis proved not to be something that punctuated the illness experience, rather the route to diagnosis was an often long and tiresome journey as opposed to a normative point on the route through the experience of illness: an experience that is reflected in other autoimmune conditions.

By contrast, more tightly regulated conditions, such as heart disease, diabetes and cancer have clearly delineated 'illness trajectories' (Nettleton, 2006) (while recognising individual experiences of that trajectory) and this is precisely what our respondents' narratives lack – 'there is no clear beginning or end; there are "no route maps" for a metaphorical journey' (Nettleton, 2006) through the autoimmune experience.

What our respondents' narratives of their diagnostic journeys patently lack is a sense of coherence and the work of Weingarten (2001) provides a useful contrasting frame of reference here. Narrative coherence, she suggests, is established by the various relationships between a narrative's plot, character roles and themes or values. In this context, patients, practitioners, carers, family members, etc., all play a part and, for many illnesses, the story's plot is well-known to all the characters. Thus, each person understands their own role and is able to anticipate events and outcomes with some degree of certainty. It is possible to examine these notions in the context of stories of diagnosis, for the experience of the respondents in our lupus research is, for the most part, in direct contrast to the notion of narrative (diagnostic) coherence; the plot of respondents' stories of diagnosis unfold in a far from coherent way. They are often confusing, the plots impenetrable and the characters unknowable and unpredictable – patients' narratives represent what we refer to as a series of vertiginous moments. As we note above, our respondents' narratives of diagnosis lack a sense of narrative coherence; their diagnostic stories do not unfold as might be expected. Indeed, for people seeking a diagnosis of lupus, and other autoimmune conditions, there is little sense of a readily accessible storyline that might guide their expectations and outcomes. It seems that each person constructs their own, very individual, story that may or may not resemble those of others with the same condition or illness experiences. This, it seems, is randomly determined by a range of unpredictable diagnostic processes, systems and individual practitioners. Even when diagnostic certainty seems imminent, its relative security can be undermined when a diagnosis is overturned or questioned.

Achieving a diagnosis of lupus, as we have demonstrated, is also somewhat serendipitous. We suggest that the bureaucratic organisation of the National Health Service in the UK is partly responsible for this; the manner in which it compartmentalises provision does not easily facilitate conversation and communication between specialists and departments, with patients in our study moving on average between three and four clinical departments. Moreover, as we demonstrate further in Chapter 3, the intellectual specialisations within medicine further exacerbate this problem, isolating practitioners in sometimes strictly ring-fenced research and practice specialisms. This point is echoed by Rosenberg (2006) in his discussion on the contested boundaries of psychiatric diagnosis in particular. He notes that diagnoses link individuals to networks of bureaucratic relationships and specialist practice. This linkage, he suggests, creates connections, but different institutional interests and practices generate conflict over policy, authority and jurisdiction. In the context of lupus, this point is particularly apposite and, while the sometimes seemingly arbitrary nature of health service provision is apparent to both clinician and patient, this situation is unlikely to change while service provision is targeted most effectively at more common conditions such as cancer and heart disease, rather than rare autoimmune conditions of which lupus is but one. Biomedical medicine has become so highly specialised and divided that it is, perhaps, difficult to reconstitute recognisably whole bodies and minds from the kaleidoscope of disparate illness experiences that people with lupus present. This is compounded in a contemporary context of tightly rationed service delivery, whereby specialist services, such as health psychology, are all too easily erased from the clinical picture. Lupus (and similar shifting conditions) fundamentally challenges biomedical medicine's trajectory towards the increasing divisions of expertise and highly specialised knowledge.

Our conceptual understanding of diagnosis is, as we have previously outlined, perhaps best described as vertiginous, drawing on the work of Doucet (2006), who invoked the conceptual notion of vertigo in the context of gender and fathering to explain where men's responses to parenting are unexpectedly at odds with gendered norms and expectations. Similarly, Young (2007) invokes the idea of vertigo to characterise the unsteadiness that permeates late modernity. Vertigo, he says, 'is the malaise of late modernity: a sense of insecurity and insubstantiality, and of uncertainty, a whiff of chaos and a fear of falling' (Young, 2007: 12). Drawing on these social conceptualisations of vertigo, we suggest that diagnosis in the context of lupus, in particular, can be usefully understood in this manner. Its presentation and symptomatology unsettle and undermine the certainty and diagnostic norms expected and promised by traditional modes of diagnosis. Adopting a modified approach to diagnosing lupus (and other uncertain conditions) may address this sense of a random experience and the concomitant sense of personal and clinical dissatisfaction that results. This would involve purposefully centring the notion of uncertainty within the doctor/patient relationship; highlighting the ways in which uncertainty operates, while exploring, with the patient, the spaces in and between the complexities of their condition. Thus, its inherent confusion and chaos could be acknowledged, examined and accepted as a requisite and anticipated part of an illness process that is to be managed, rather than ignored and/or expelled from the disease equation. To this end, Goldstein Jutel and Dew (2014: 230) have developed a diagnostic mnemonic, CLASSIFY, which they hope will be of value to medical practitioners.

**C** – certainty (how important is it/its absence?)
**L** – label (who benefits and why?)
**A** – alternate (are there alternative belief/healing systems that have a role?)
**S** – social context (what is the patient's context and is it relevant?)
**S** – stigma (is it going to cause stigma and how?)
**I** – information (sources and provision)
**F** – financial (who is paying for treatment and what are the implications?)
**Y** – you (classify yourself)

Centring uncertainty in this way would, of course, require a modified understanding of the clinical encounter from both the patient's and clinician's perspective. More problematic, perhaps, is the fact that this renegotiation of the purpose and utility of diagnosis would demand a new language – a semantics of ambiguity and uncertainty that might enable a redefined dialogue to take place, not only within the clinical encounter, but also in the various social spaces that the diagnosis of illness occupies. At present, without a means to define and linguistically delineate the experience of illness (without a definitive diagnosis) it seems we are lost in our attempts to explain what is wrong. Further, the socially sanctioned access to the 'benefits' of illness (medical resources, workplace benefits, social approbation, etc.) are, at present, difficult, if not impossible, to access without recourse to a defining and explanatory label.

In the context of lupus, however, there may be a space in which to at least partially achieve these aims. The clinical markers for lupus have changed over the years, reflecting the varying paradigms of any respective era. It has, for example, been classified as a dermatological condition, a disease of the immune system and, more recently, a genetic disorder (Stockl, 2007). The clinical criteria governing the diagnosis of lupus are, thus, mutable, as more is known about the condition and the ways in which responses to it are regulated and mediated. Rather than perceiving lupus as a discrete disease entity, perhaps it would be more fruitful to think of it as a syndrome or spectrum, although we are mindful of the fact that one of the ironic effects of a condition being referred to as a 'syndrome' is that it may then be regarded as contested, as in the case of IBS, for example. Diagnostic criteria could then be less tightly drawn and would give space, within the boundaries of the condition, to experience the mildest incarnations of lupus, through to the most serious and life-threatening. This might allow a degree of diagnostic freedom and clinical autonomy for both patient and practitioner alike.

Our example of the diagnostic process in Lupus illustrates the ways in which it operates to underpin the power of professionals and the range of vested interests that the classification and naming of illness experience serves. Jutel (2013) likens diagnosis to being in a crowded room in which different participants (and processes) jostle for position and authority – the room comprises values and norms, patient advocacy groups, social movements, information, authorities, industries, belief systems, professional hierarchies, funding and finances, and technologies – all competing and playing a part in the process of either acquiring or determining a diagnosis. Bell (2014), in a study of infertility, similarly draws our attention to the racial, gendered and class dimensions of diagnosis. It also demonstrates the variety of ways in which people that are ill may, with the help of new technologies and interactive fora, challenge the operation of power by the medical profession and take back some control of their illness experience. Moreover, these fora and new technologies may also offer respite from the uncertainty of the diagnostic process and the seeming inadequacies of some clinical encounters.[2]

The concept of 'embodied doubt, a feature of contemporary life' (Nettleton, 2006: 1169) situates our analysis of our respondents' diagnostic journeys, as does the concomitant notion of diagnostic doubt. It is the confluence of symptomatic, physical, clinical and technological uncertainty that explains both the time it can take to generate a diagnosis and the changed and changing nature of the diagnostic process itself. This process is characterised by fluidity, rather than certainty – indeed, as we have suggested, it might usefully be referred to as diagnostic vertigo. Respondents' experiences thus reflect and refract and embody the uncertainty characteristic of late modernity (Bauman, 1993). The difficulties they experience in acquiring a name for their illness and the ways in which that naming does, for some, eventually take place, is a reflection of the ways in which, 'the relations with codified expertise and everyday life can be tenuous' (Nettleton, 2006: 1176). The act/process of diagnosis in lupus is a very particular example of this, as it is a certain condition with a most uncertain aetiology, course and outcome. Indeed, the challenges of diagnosing lupus and other similarly diffuse autoimmune conditions help illuminate a complex interplay of issues that extend far beyond the borders of the disease.

## Notes

1  See Chapter 3 for a discussion on the iatrogenic effects of navigating health services.
2  Although arguably pre-diagnostic screening resulting in predictive diagnosis or indeed being determined as 'pre-ill' on the basis of certain characteristics unsettles the diagnostic process further still (Salter et al., 2011).

## References

Anderson, W. and Mackay, I.R. (2014) *Intolerant Bodies: A Short History of Autoimmunity*. Baltimore: John Hopkins University Press.

Bauman, Z. (2000) *Liquid Modernity*. Cambridge: Polity Press.

Bell, A. V. (2014) 'Diagnostic Diversity: The Role of Social Class in Diagnostic Experiences of Infertility'. *Sociology of Health & Illness* 36(4): 516–530.

Brown, P. (1995) 'Naming and Framing: The Social Construction of Diagnosis and Illness'. *Journal of Health and Social Behavior* 35: 34–52.

Brown, P., Lyson, M. and Jenkins, T. (2009) 'From Diagnosis to Social Diagnosis'. *Social Science and Medicine* 73(6): 939–943.

Corbin, J. and Strauss, A. (1985) 'Managing Chronic Illness at Home: Three Lines of Work'. *Qualitative Sociology* 8(3): 224–247.

Doucet, A. (2006) *Do Men Mother?* Toronto: University of Toronto Press.

Dumit, J. (2006) 'Illnesses You Have to Fight to Get: Facts as Forces in Uncertain, Emergent Illnesses'. *Social Science & Medicine* 62(3): 577–590.

Goldstein Jutel, A. (2014) 'When the Penny Drops: Diagnosis and the Transformative Moment'. In A. Goldstein Jutel and K. Dew (eds), *Social Issues in Diagnosis: An Introduction for Students and Clinicians*. Baltimore: Johns Hopkins University Press.

Goldstein Jutel, A. and Dew, K. (eds) (2014) *Social Issues in Diagnosis: An Introduction for Students and Clinicians*. Baltimore: Johns Hopkins University Press.

Jutel, A. (2009) 'Sociology of Diagnosis: A Preliminary Review'. *Sociology of Health & Illness* 31(2): 278–299.

Jutel, A. (2011) *Putting a Name to It: Diagnosis in Contemporary Society*. Baltimore, MD: Johns Hopkins University Press.

Jutel, A. (2013) *The Sociology of Diagnosis*. Seminar presented as part of the ESRC series *The Role of Diagnosis in Health & Wellbeing: A Social Science Perspective on the Social, Economic and Political Costs and Consequences of Diagnosis*, www.youtube.com/watch?v=ROOTtssUIDc (accessed 23 February 2014).

Lupus UK (2012) *Diagnosis*, www.lupusuk.org.uk/what-is-lupus/diagnosis (accessed 12 December 2012).

Mendelson, C. (2006) 'Managing a Medically and Socially Complex Life: Women Living with Lupus'. *Qualitative Health Research* 16(7): 982–997.

Mendelson, C. (2009) 'Diagnosis: A Liminal State for Women Living With Lupus'. *Health Care for Women International* 30: 390–407.

Miles, A. (2013) *Living with Lupus: Women and Chronic Illness in Ecuador*. Austin: University of Texas Press.

Mol, A. (2002) *The Body Multiple: Ontology in Medical Practice*. Durham, NC, and London: Duke University Press.

Nettleton, S. (2004) 'The Emergence of E-scaped Medicine?' *Sociology* 38(4): 661–679.

Nettleton, S. (2006) '"I Just Want Permission to be Ill": Towards a Sociology of Medically Unexplained Symptoms'. *Social Science & Medicine* 62: 1167–1178.

Novas, C. and Rose, N. (2000) 'Genetic Risk and the Birth of the Somatic Individual'. *Economy and Society* 29(4): 485–513.

Olson, R. and Abeysinghe, S. (2014) 'None of the Above: Uncertainty and Diagnosis'. In, A. Goldstein Jutel and K. Dew (eds), *Social Issues in Diagnosis: An Introduction for Students and Clinicians*. Baltimore: Johns Hopkins University Press.

Parsons, T. (1951) *The Social System*. New York: The Free Press.

Rosenberg, C. E. (2006) 'Contested Boundaries: Psychiatry, Disease, and Diagnosis'. *Perspectives in Biology and Medicine* 49(3): 407–424.

Salter, C., Howe, A., McDaid, L., Blacklock, J., Lenaghan, E. and Shepstone, L. (2011) 'Risk, Significance and Biomedicalisation of a New Population: Older Women's Experience of Osteoporosis Screening'. *Social Science & Medicine* 73: 808–815.

Sayce, L. (1999) *From Psychiatric Patient to Citizen: Overcoming Discrimination and Social Exclusion*. London: Palgrave Macmillan.

Sontag, S. (2001) *Illness as Metaphor and AIDS and its Metaphors*. London: Picador.

Stockl, A. (2007) 'Complex Syndromes, Ambivalent Diagnosis, and Existential Uncertainty: The Case of Systemic Lupus Erythematosus (SLE)'. *Social Science & Medicine* 65: 1549–1559.

Stoller, P. (2004) *Stranger in the Village of the Sick: A Memoir of Cancer, Sorcery and Healing*. Boston: Beacon Press.

Weingarten, K. (2001) *Working with the Stories of Women's Lives*. Adelaide: Dulwich Centre Publications.

Young, J. (2007) *The Vertigo of Late Modernity*. London: Sage.

# 3 Patients, professionals and the clinical encounter – making the connections

As Chapter 2 has already demonstrated, the clinical encounter[1] and its complex dynamics sits, often uneasily, at the heart of the illness experience – in the context of the autoimmune experience, diagnosis is simply the beginning (and part) of what will prove to be a lifelong relationship with healthcare providers. The social, political and policy context in which this relationship occurs and the ways in which power and authority are enacted (on both sides of the encounter) are its defining features that can colour, and often determine, a person's trajectory through their illness journey.

The relationship is at once easily understood by all actors in the clinical relationship, while, at the same time, being a complex interplay of social, political, scientific and psychological processes that come together to constitute the clinical encounter. This encounter occurs, most often, at times of acute vulnerability and distress for patients and, given the pressures of time and resources that are increasingly evident in contemporary healthcare, it can be variously constrained and time-limited, meaning that it is not always possible for practitioners to affect a reasonable system of communication with patients, which can be frustrating for both.

As noted above, however, at the heart of the relationship between patient and practitioner lies an implicit understanding of the roles each person is expected to play in addition to the narratives, plots and themes that have been both predetermined and clearly defined over centuries of medical intervention. Historically, the physician has 'known best' how to interpret, understand and treat a patient's malady, but the march of science and technology has, paradoxically, undermined both public faith in medicine and the clinical certainty that medical professionals have traditionally enjoyed. The pressure to work in person-centred ways, involving patients (who, for their part, have far greater access to readily available information about their symptoms/condition/treatment than ever before) in the diagnosis and treatment of illness and decision-making in that context, coupled with an increasingly cynical consumer base that has the power to both influence and judge clinical practice, has the propensity to generate profound existential uncertainty for both the purveyors and consumers of contemporary healthcare. Indeed, the uncertainty that is evident in many of our respondents' narratives is of a particularly ironic nature given that medical science promises so much in the context of illuminating the aetiology, epidemiology and, indeed, the epistemology of illness. Moreover, given the major advances recent years have generated in terms of detection, diagnosis and treatment for all manner of physical illnesses, the public, in turn, has come to expect things from medicine that it was never going to be able (and was not necessarily designed) to offer. That is, the demand for medical certainty has never been greater, yet access to it, despite – and in some cases because of – the advances in clinical medicine, is increasingly limited. The public expect answers to medical questions (many of which they now have some degree of access to themselves), which the medical profession is unable to supply.

In this chapter, we explore patients' experiences of the clinical encounter in the context of lupus, focusing on their developing patient identities in an increasingly consumer/provider-orientated healthcare system and the medical profession's response in a resource-hungry, time-limited and often poorly staffed context. We further develop some of the themes introduced in Chapter 2 and focus, in particular, on the enactment of medical authority, and patients' various responses to it, in the context of autoimmune disease. Our analysis, however, extends to the wider medical world beyond the clinic, to explore the ways in which the construction of health services more generally might impact upon the autoimmune patient experience. Three critical themes emerge from our respondents' experiences of the clinical encounter (and are reflected in some other autoimmune conditions). The first relates to the notion of the patient as a consumer in twenty-first-century healthcare contexts, the second, the necessity for those with autoimmune conditions to engage with multiple clinical specialisms and departments (a continuation of their diagnostic journey) and, third, the sometimes iatrogenic consequences of negotiating these complex systems in a context of shrinking resources. We also refer, briefly, to experiences from the opposite side of the clinical encounter.

There is a general tradition of understanding and framing the clinical encounter, in the sociological and psychological literature, which speaks very clearly to power relations – that is, in the social and political contexts in which it occurs (Giddens, 1991; Werner and Malterud, 2003; Young, 2007). While this body of scholarship is one in which our own work is broadly situated, we purposefully focus here on the clinical encounter in relation to the specific experience of lupus (and other autoimmune conditions where they pertain more generally).

We do this because, to date, in the relevant literature, individuals' experiences and narratives reflect the specificities of the particular area of the body affected by their condition (see, for example, Mol, 2002). What we have found during our examination of lupus (which is reflected in other autoimmune conditions such as scleroderma and multiple sclerosis) is, of course, the whole body multi/system involvement and high prevalence of co-morbidities. We stress that while we appreciate that a cardiovascular problem, for example, affects the whole person and their wider social context, it would be unlikely that a patient diagnosed with a cardiovascular condition would find themselves involved in any specialism other than cardiology. They would not, in all likelihood, be referred to a gastroenterologist, a dermatologist or even a psychiatrist in a search for the clinical meaning and management of their symptoms. But, as we have demonstrated earlier, this is a common experience for people with lupus. As such, this condition is a multisystem/multidiscipline experience. Through a specific focus on lupus, we demonstrate the complexities of living as a 'patchwork patient', where little clinical support may be forthcoming in (to further the needlework analogy) stitching the pieces of the clinical patchwork together. We frame our discussion of the patchwork patient in light of a more general discussion on the policy context within which the clinical encounter has unfolded in the recent past. It follows from this that we identify a critical need for clinical and social connectivity, which itself is somewhat ironic in the context of a connective tissue disease.[2] We would argue that it is here that professions not ordinarily seen at the forefront of the clinical response to lupus and other autoimmune conditions may have a critical role to play.

## Unpacking the clinical encounter in lupus: producers and consumers in health

Recent decades have seen a number of unprecedented shifts in the ways in which healthcare is provided by professionals and experienced by the public. Social and political change and the advent of web-based information sharing and consumption has generated 'an unsettling of the consumer-organisational interface' that has 'forced the renegotiation of respective roles and power relationships' (Laing et al., 2010: 9). The 'patient', traditionally a vessel through and onto which professional expertise and power was enacted, has now assumed a more proactive, assertive and informed perspective that actively challenges biomedical authority and power. In some contexts this is very much welcomed and, in others, actively resisted.

> The patient as consumer desires to produce his/her own medico-administrative identity through interaction with physicians, nurses and technologies. This has contributed to the diminution of medical authority as well as increased expectations (and incidences of dissatisfaction) regarding the quality of service. Yet these post-modern currents inevitably collide with the more intractable, modernist features of the medico-administrative system.
>
> (Thompson, 2003: 103)

Laing et al. (2010) suggest that the tensions inherent in this newly framed personal and professional milieu are discernible in the ways in which the clinical encounter has shifted away from those characterised by deference and compliance on the part of the patient to those which are more redolent of notions such as patient centeredness.

In the UK, it is the personalisation agenda, or 'care transition' as Taylor and Bury (2007) refer to it, that is, perhaps, most indicative of this shift – it is a key concept that underpins the changes to the ways in which health and social care is provided and the ways in which patients variously experience them (while the notion of personalisation is invoked most often in the context of social – rather than health – care, we introduce it here to describe a particular ideological focus in health services). This personalisation initiative, founded on the principles of empowerment, choice, involvement and decision-making, has been the principal driver behind other policy initiatives that reflect a political will focused on generating a new patient/service user personae in the modernised NHS, which incorporates a range of rights and responsibilities that may or may not, depending on the patient's capabilities and proclivities, be embraced by the public (see, for example, Department of Health (1999; 2004a; 2004b; NHS Executive, 1998). Most evident in the provision of social care services, the personalisation agenda is, nonetheless, indicative of a range of government policy initiatives that have, at their heart, the concept of the patient as consumer. It represents an ideological shift in both policy and practice that claims to put the person at the centre of intervention and here we use it to describe and illuminate the current focus in the NHS in the UK on the patient and their healthcare experience.[3]

Central to the notion of personalisation, and other more explicitly health focused policy initiatives, has been some acknowledgement of the patient as expert in their own experience and, by definition, manager of their own health outcomes. This, it could be argued, reflects a postmodern exemplification of the notions of justice, respect and partnership (NHS Modernisation Agency, 2004), which was exemplified in the Expert Patient Programme (EPP), a government initiative, established in the UK in 2001 (Department of Health, 2001), which was formulated in response to the work of Kate Lorig in the USA, who had developed a programme of self-management and efficacy for people living with chronic illness (in this case, specifically, arthritis). The programme involved the delivery (by healthcare professionals) of self-management training that centred on an 'anecdotal vision of the "active patient"' (Laing et al., 2010) that was implicitly underpinned by a biomedical presumption of capacity and motivation to undertake goal-oriented tasks expected by healthcare professionals (Greenhalgh, 2009). The discourse of the expert patient was founded on the notion that each person living with illness knows best what hinders and helps them manage the day to day realties of ill-health most effectively. It represented the introduction of a wider and long-lasting policy trend in health and social care in the UK towards self-management and self-care with ever-increasing involvement of carers, family and digital technologies (Taylor and Bury, 2007). We invoke the EPP here, as a useful mechanism through which to explore power and change in the clinical encounter.

One of the respondents in our lupus study had been actively involved in the programme:

> **Corrine:** I've been on a couple of courses that have helped a lot. One was run by the community health psychologist and the other was the Expert Patient Programme (EPP). The best thing about both courses was that it allowed us [the chronically ill patients] to discuss our illnesses and all the baggage that comes with them. We laughed, cried and helped each other.

Corrine's story explicates the positive benefits of the programme, which are, for this person, perhaps not what policymakers had intended. For them, the benefits of this shift were, theoretically, twofold – potentially improved outcomes for consumers of health and care provision and greater efficiency and effectiveness of service provision (Laing et al., 2010). Indeed, patients' improved connectedness with their own healthcare has shown to bring about significant improvements in healthcare outcomes and the potential advantages of joined up decision-making are clear – better healthcare outcomes, better compliance with treatment regimes, better informed and more satisfied patients, etc. With access to previously unavailable information (in the technological age) and the various opportunities to engage more fully (and critically) in the clinical relationship, the patient becomes less a passive vessel for medical intervention and, arguably, more the 'proto-professional' we referred to in Chapter 2 (Novas and Rose, 2000) in the clinical relationship and the illness journey. The patient, in this context, becomes, theoretically, a participant in the clinical process, which in turn creates a 'therapeutic alliance' between patient and practitioner in which the patient must be 'skilled, prudent and active' and, as a partner in this alliance, must also take responsibility for the successful outcome of the collaboration (Stockl, 2007: 1557). This responsibility presupposes both a willingness and ability to engage in collaboration from both patient and practitioner. To do so, however, demands a palpable shift in focus from a paternalistic medical model and a passive patient role.

As we have noted above, the EPP was emblematic of this ideological shift and, while it was premised on the notion of educating the patient in the techniques of self-management, it has, seemingly, transcended the boundaries of its official status. That is, it has provided benefits to patients that were not envisaged (or, perhaps desired) by service providers. Further, it is, at once, emblematic of changes in the ways in which patients are expected to operate in the context of a shift towards more person-centred clinical practice, more broadly, but also provides a critical challenge to professions that have traditionally enjoyed the positive balance of power in the clinical relationship.

> We know from reading the press and listening to the debate that when doctors come across the term 'expert patient' they hear different things. For the chief medical officer, expert patients are 'people who have the confidence, skills, information and knowledge to play a central role in the management of life with chronic diseases'. The suspicion is that for many doctors, the expert patient of the imagination is the one clutching a sheaf of printouts from the internet demanding a particular treatment that is unproved, manifestly unsuitable, astronomically expensive, or all three.
>
> (Shaw and Baker, 2004: 723)

The EPP, therefore, means very different things to different people depending upon the context in which they are operating, but the ideological basis on which it was developed remains clear and influential. As Taylor and Bury (2007: 41) argue, 'although to many NHS staff the EPP may at present seem to be of only marginal importance, the thinking upon which it is based is likely to influence the future delivery of all high-quality medical, pharmaceutical and nursing care'.

So, while some patients may, indeed, embody the confident, informed and assertive role outlined in initiatives such as EPP, the prospect of having to relinquish power in this context appears to come more easily to some practitioners than others. For, in the context of autoimmune conditions, this is not simply a case of sharing information and decision-making with the patient. As we have previously suggested, this entails also embracing uncertainty and making evident the imprecise nature of the medical knowledge that underpins autoimmune conditions (and many others). This, in itself, is very much at odds with the paternalistic model of healthcare both patients and practitioners are more familiar with subscribing to and operating within.

Uncertainty, however, is an inescapable feature of all medical practice; the ways in which patients can now access information and knowledge demands a degree of reflection from practitioners and the relinquishing of some of the power or, at the very least, the practice of certainty, medicine has traditionally enjoyed. This, however, would inevitably demystify and simultaneously make explicit that uncertainty; a process that may be threatening and, arguably, deeply undermining for practitioners – despite the fact that uncertainty and clinical doubt are facts of medical life, they are rarely fully acknowledged or actively engaged. Uncertainty is a threat to the trusted structures of the clinical relationship (as we shall see in the narratives we present in this chapter) in that acknowledging clinical uncertainty is to admit the intellectual and practice specific boundaries of medicine and, in so doing, challenge and potentially undermine medical authority and medicine's a priori knowledge of the body and its machinations.

> For sharing uncertainties requires a willingness to admit ignorance about benefits and risks; to profess to the existence of alternatives, each with its own known and unknown consequences; to eschew one single authoritative recommendation; to consider carefully how to present uncertainties so that patients will not become overwhelmed by the information they are required to know; and to explore the crucial question of how much uncertainty physicians themselves can tolerate without compromising their effectiveness as healers.

> (Katz, 1987: 209)

It is, of course, the interpersonal context that actually drives the experience shared by patients and practitioners and where the impact of new ideologies of care, of patient choice and patient-centredness, are at their most transparent. It remains to be seen whether the prevailing political and social will is, however, evident in day-to-day practice in health and social care situations or whether prevailing paternalistic, biomedical philosophies and ideologies of care endure. As will become evident, our data strongly suggest the latter and, as Laing et al. (2010) note, while actively involving people in their own healthcare decision-making arguably leads to better long-term health outcomes, this model simultaneously places increasing demands upon patients to be resourced (socially and financially), informed, active and motivated in the context of their self-management, something that not all people are willing or able to do. Empowered participation in the clinical encounter presupposes a degree of social power that, if limited, may curtail the ability to fully engage in new processes and ways of working.

For professionals too, there are difficulties inherent in these new approaches, particularly in the context of working in partnership with patients. We would suggest that biomedical power is not something easily displaced by politically driven initiatives – that is to say that paternalistic healthcare practice is intractably embedded in the expectations and presumptions that underpin the relationships that are enacted in our healthcare systems. Our data, to which we now turn further, would certainly seem to clearly underline this point.

## Confident consumers

Evidence of the interpersonal and social power to which we refer above and the assertiveness and confidence of the newly informed consumer demanded by politically driven healthcare initiatives was amply evident in our data. Informed and assertive, the following respondents demonstrate a palpable confidence in both their ability to communicate their needs and expectations and a non-compromising approach to addressing the difficulties lupus presents them with. While articulate and assertive, what their narratives also indicate is the fact that they seem to have been 'lucky' to have professionals involved in their care who are prepared to work in collaboration with them – that is, in a person-centred way.

Penny and the other respondents below have positioned themselves confidently at the centre of their care, undertaking quasi-clinical work and the micromanagement of their illness. Their approach to the self-management of their condition is indicative of the type of patient who is motivated and able to engage on level terms with the professionals involved in their care. They are the archetypal proto-professional patients.

> **Penny:** My GP practice and INR nurse at the practice are great, my GP didn't know a lot about lupus when I joined the practice but I gave them literature and he went away and investigated lupus, they're so supportive and helpful, I try not to visit unless absolutely necessary (the place is full of sick people, I tell them). They know if I turn up there I'm very unwell. I see my INR nurse every four months to synchronise and check my machine, I'm self-testing as my INR is unstable and I have to adjust doses of warfarin. If I have any problems I only have to phone in and I'll either be seen or get advice over the phone. I also have clexane to take if my INR drops too far out of range… I find I'm able to be very involved in my treatment.

In order to communicate the degree of in-depth knowledge Penny has, and that which underpins her ability to understand and manage her condition, she fruitfully employs the clinical language of lupus. Penny is diagnosed with antiphospholipid syndrome and the INR – international normalised ratio – is a measurement used to monitor the effectiveness of warfarin (an anti-coagulant). Similarly, Belle, who also has antiphospholipid syndrome in addition to lupus, works with a team of professionals to coordinate a complex range of individual clinical relationships, the centre of which she confidently occupies.

> **Belle:** My experience with my consultants (I have loads wrong with me) is wonderful. I am under [NHS Trust] and have absolutely no problems whatsoever

(I probably shouldn't say this in case something goes wrong!) The consultants work with me, my lifestyle and lupus and I also have control over my drugs and how to adjust my warfarin for my INR. My treatment is based on both parties being happy and working together to ensure that I have the best possible life that I can lead with this devastating illness. I generally see my haematologist every four to six weeks and my other consultants on a six-month basis or more if necessary. The lupus specialist, in my opinion, is the least involved. I currently see him on a six-monthly basis but this was on my insistence as he only wants to see a lupus patient yearly. As far as I'm concerned that just isn't good enough. A lupus consultant should be involved on a three- to six-month (or more) basis, not yearly.

As for my GP, they are also good although not so experienced. I have a working relationship with them but I find that they can be quite skittish when it comes to some of my treatments (I am heavily medicated) and in particular my INR levels (I have a very volatile INR). I keep them as up-to-date as possible and try to see my regular GP on a six- to eight-week basis to keep them involved, although they do get regular letters from my consultants.

Similarly, for Andrew, an assertiveness and a confidence in the right to medical attention was often brought to bear in situations where others might fare less well. Often acutely ill, Andrew brought his business acumen and assertiveness to clinical encounters. He is a man who exudes confidence in his right to be heard and brought this confidence to the relationships he shares with professionals.

**Andrew:** I suppose for me, I mean my whole career was based around questioning and challenging… You know, because I was sorting businesses that were in trouble, and I was sorting out entirely new ways of doing business, you know, so yeah… that's how I've spent my life and I suppose that's been an advantage really in terms of remaining on this planet. You can talk to your doctors, which I think is incredibly important, I think if there's one thing about anybody with a chronic illness or a lifelong illness is they don't talk to their doctors, they just take what the doctor says and okay doctor, that's fine, and I don't believe you should do that, I think you should use a modicum of intelligence and ask them about your condition, ask them about the medication that you're on or they're suggesting you go on and do your own research into that and find out what the possible implications of that are and also, more importantly, talk to them about the future, you know, and is there anything you can do to alleviate the problem and, and, and perhaps slow down the progression of what it is?… that to me is very important.

I never have short consultants' visits… I don't care how much time they've allotted, whether it's ten minutes or twenty minutes, it'll take as much time as I need… and nobody's ever looked at their watch and said to me 'roll up son… time's up'. I have had a few dirty looks sometimes when I come out from the people who are sat in the waiting rooms.

What these excerpts demonstrate is, as we have said, the confident, informed approach taken by some of our respondents, but what they also indicate is the amount of energy these people, in particular, were required to expend ensuring that the care they received was optimal. This confidence and the ability to assert the right to joined up, competent care was not, however, something enjoyed by everyone we spoke to.

**Moira:** My first GP kept telling me I was getting growing pains, migraines, anaemia, eczema, stress (what does an 11-year-old have to be stressed about?), but these weren't connected and I shouldn't worry about them. Eventually, it was put down to a virus and I felt as though I was wasting my time going. The last time I saw him before we moved practices I had a discoid-type rash on my back that exactly followed the line of the tops I'd been wearing at the time in the middle of summer. I got fobbed off again, given some E45 and that was it.

We moved practices shortly after that and just before I had my first real flare. My GP there started off wonderfully and tested me for SLE very quickly but soon lost interest when all of my bloods kept coming back normal. She kept telling me I was stressed. I switched GPs within the practice and I really haven't regretted it considering that this one seems to be the only GP who has ever believed me. She told me recently that she suspected SLE the very first time I saw her, which was a full two years before diagnosis. She will admit that she doesn't know a lot about it, but has always been willing to go away and check, she's not afraid to admit she doesn't know what more she can do and always listens to what I've got to say, even if it is a pile of crap. She really has been a great support and I can only wish that every GP will be half as good as she's been.

Consultants are another story. My first rheumatologist was awful, didn't speak to me, didn't listen to me and didn't really do a lot for me. She discharged me twice, first time saying that I was post-viral, the second after telling me I had a butterfly rash, was photosensitive and treated me for Raynaud's. She told me that I'd be back to normal if I started to swim, which I did, and it only made me worse. My current rheumatologist is far better than that and he actually has time to listen to me and, more importantly, answer those questions that no one else can.

I've also had a pretty bad experience with a gastroenterologist, which is along the lines of not being believed. It got so bad that on my first appointment with him I sat in protest for over an hour to try and get him to see things from my perspective. The one thing I will say about him was that he was the only one before diagnosis who thought I had the start of a connective tissue disease, so he must have eventually believed me.

The only people hospital-related, apart from my rheumatologist, who has treated me as a person and not a list of symptoms were the nurse who inserted my pH probe and my dietician. Both are the only ones who have had time to talk about things other than what's going on with me physically and that really did make all the difference. Sometimes it's nice to be talked to as a person and not a patient, something that I keep telling my medical student friends.

The distinction between Moira's dual identity as person and patient identified in this narrative is an interesting and purposeful one. One's personhood is, she would suggest, compromised in the clinical relationship – further evidence of the imbalance of power in this context. Her account points clearly to the necessity to engage with the whole person in the clinic, rather than the more easily abstracted specificities of the disease process. The lack of regard, communication and simple organisation referred to by Moira was not an uncommon experience for our respondents. For Cora, her assertiveness, unlike the people quoted above, did not result in increased clinical attentiveness, rather, it compounded already difficult relationships. In addition, she goes further, to identify a point at which her identity was fundamentally undermined by her relationships with professionals – she was perceived to be, she states, a 'non-person', surely anathema to a clinical project designed to underscore a person-centred approach to practice.

**Cora:** I was diagnosed with a number of rheumatic illnesses before I was diagnosed with lupus about 15 years ago. Since then, it has been a total roller-coaster of treatment, about four to five years into my diagnosis, my rheumy retired and I was allocated another one, that's when everything started going downhill.

My new rheumy could not get his act together, my blood tests kept getting lost or he didn't bother doing any. Eventually, three years ago, a result from an ANA test came back borderline on the positive side, and he told me that I was cured, ha! So, all my medication was stopped.

At the same time as my rheumy changing, I had to move house because of my decreasing mobility, had to get a new GP. They did not understand a thing about lupus. Every time I went to them with a new or persistent symptom, they would just say it was the lupus and there was nothing they could do about it instead of investigating. Take my thyroid for instance, it took three years for them to refer me to a specialist, had to have half of it taken out because it was so badly swollen that it was strangling slowly and my oxygen level was so low that they had to oxygenate me for 48 hours. I am almost positive that I should be on thyroxin, but hey, who cares!

I have had to fight long and hard for the doctors to give me my diagnosis back so that I can go back on my medication. Thankfully now, I think I might have bagged a sympathetic rheumy, he has given me a steroid injection and said that if it works, he will put me back on plaquenil. The steroid injection did work, sadly, it has now worn off but going back to the rheumy next week. What really hurts more than anything else, it is how much of a non-person the medical profession can make you feel. I have been struck off the register of two GPs' surgeries because of my insistence for treatment and a second opinion.

I don't have any support and I think it is the fact that I started asking the question 'How can you medical people just accept the fact that one rheumatologist says that I am cured of an incurable illness based on the result of one blood test, which isn't even negative?' Also, I kept asking for a different rheumy, I think in the end they just got so fed up of me that they changed the rheumy to shut me up. I am so glad they did though, I went to the new rheumy today and he has put me back on plaquenil, given me another steroid injection to give the tablets chance to work and, obviously, my diagnosis back. He says that the lupus is active but only mildly; I'd hate to have it bad! He is also sending me to the physio to see if they can help.

I forgot to tell you that while all this was happening, the GP sent me to the psychiatrist because he said it was all in my head, the psychiatrist said there was nothing wrong with me apart from being in extreme pain.

What these purposefully lengthy narratives demonstrate is a critical shift away from the vertiginous experience of diagnosis, which has been demonstrated to be a common experience for all our respondents, towards an experience that, for some, assumes a freefall trajectory and, for others, a journey that is characterised by an increasing sense of self and externally imposed control and management. To extend the analogy, following diagnosis, some people experience freefall, while others are lucky to be provided with clinical parachutes that cushion and guide their journey through the turbulence of the illness air currents. The nature of their experience, however, is fundamentally mediated by the seemingly arbitrary nature of the clinical encounter and the ways in which a satisfactory patient experience is founded, to a profound degree, on the vagaries of individual professionals' interpersonal skills and their willingness to allow patients the opportunity to fully engage in the experience of their own illness. This, what would seem to be a most basic right, demands, however, that professional's historically sanctioned reliance on clinical paternalism is relinquished along with developing an acknowledgement and awareness of the need to work with rather than around the patient. This is less public policy and more, perhaps, an unintended outcome of demographic change, a rise in the numbers of people diagnosed with long-term conditions and the advancement of knowledge (without a corresponding rise in public health related expenditure) (Taylor and Bury, 2007).

The fragmentation that we would argue results from this situation reflects, and is compounded by, the increasing specialisation in clinical medicine and the subsequent micro-partition of healthcare provision that has resulted in people's experience of care being increasingly disaggregated, as they are referred to and between multiple clinical departments in a search of both diagnosis and the management of prognosis. In these clinical specialities, people's experiences suggest that there is a tendency to adopt a 'head in the sand' approach to connected care – that is, clinical specialisms turn increasingly inwards as the science of medicine does the same. As a result, the physical body is gradually decontextualised and arguably dehumanised, it is deconstructed and compartmentalised into increasingly minute components that become difficult to reconstitute into human wholes. It would seem that professionals, perhaps understandably under these circumstances and the pressures of working in resource limited contexts, find it difficult to perceive – to actually *see* – a whole person in this context. Second, for people with lupus – who may find themselves first at the GP, then the dermatologist, then the cardiologist, nephrologist or rheumatologist – the resulting communication difficulties (for both patients and other professionals) can exacerbate the 'patchwork' nature of their clinical encounters (Gardner et al., 2011; Mol, 2002), which can prove to be frustrating in the extreme.

**Amanda:** Even the best professionals are battling against the tide, in terms of time, cost and availability of services. Because of this, care is always fragmented and there is no one person who brings practical help, medical knowledge and psychological support all together.

Mol's (2002) ethnographic work on the ontology of care practices provides a compelling illustration of the patchwork metaphor. She demonstrated the multiple ways in which a single diagnosis, atherosclerosis, could be experienced, read and treated and provides examples of these multiplicities. In atherosclerosis, the arteries in the legs become thickened and clogged with plaques of fatty substances, or atheromas, which narrow the arteries potentially causing a blockage. Symptoms can include angina, claudication (pain and cramping in the lower leg during exercise) and, possible heart attack and stroke. Mol (2002) demonstrated that, although atherosclerosis is a single diagnosis with a clearly defined symptomatology and treatment approach, the ways in which it is understood will be different in the various locales within a hospital. The pathologist, for example refers to the *sound* of atherosclerosis in a dead body, the auditory exemplification of the condition 'when the resident takes her scissors to cut the aorta, she warns me: "Listen! Yeah! Do you hear that? There's your atherosclerosis". I hear it. A cracking sound. Calcification' (Mol, 2002: 125). In another area of the hospital, perhaps the outpatients' department, the condition is read as the suffering caused to the patient, while, in another, the laboratory, for instance, it is abstracted into the various ways in which the constituent chemicals in the blood can work to generate the fatty deposits that are the cause of the problem. One diagnosis, then, is multiple and the hospital houses this multiplicity of readings and responses. In order to effectively treat the patient, these different readings need to be communicated and coordinated, something that, Mol suggests, can be particularly challenging to operationalise. After Mol (2002) and Gardner et al. (2011), we would refer to lupus as a patchwork diagnosis and people with lupus as 'patchwork patients'. Prior to diagnosis, in particular, their condition is diffuse and unknown and, as such, they are at the mercy of the various clinical departments within the hospital setting. As we have demonstrated in Chapter 2, here people are very much dependent upon where they are first referred (this, as we have shown, can have profound effect on the speed and accuracy of diagnosis). This may be a rheumatologist, but is just as likely to be a dermatologist or cardiologist, who are all apt to read the person's symptoms through their specialist lens. If the symptoms do not necessarily 'fit' their own clinical world view, our respondents' narratives suggest that the possibility of any one consultant taking the time to try to piece together the jigsaw of the lupus experience is unlikely. Post-diagnosis, the situation does not necessarily change, as the systemic nature of the condition means that people will move between multiple clinical specialisms as new symptoms arise and require investigation and treatment, their treatment elsewhere in the hospital can be perceived as a seemingly unrelated issue. In these piecemeal situations, the person's body is read differently depending on which specialist department they find themselves referred to. Lupus can present as a patchwork of clinically unrelated problems (that are only reconstituted in the whole, perhaps, by the patient themselves). People with lupus are thus impelled to become their own care managers and coordinators and develop their own care plan, there is no one else to do the job and this coordinating role places an additional strain on an already limited supply of physical and existential resources. As Mol (2002) suggests, in the context of atherosclerosis, the patchwork that makes up the various problems associated with the condition are not easily married up but, if care is to be effective, they must be. The patchwork Mol refers to is the linking together of the disparate data and practices that will allow this to happen. What people with lupus would, perhaps, benefit from is a person or system (other than themselves) that is capable of creating a recognisable and useable patchwork from their disparate strands of symptoms, experiences, clinical data, specialist departments and different consultants' opinions.

> **Wendy:** I feel very alone with lupus… I have rarely gone to a GP, as on the odd occasion I have I am told its 'normal' to have this ill feeling (or whatever ailment I have gone with) with lupus. Even on specialist appointments, everything is rushed, nothing is explained. On one occasion I was very ill (barely able to walk) and told that everything was okay as the lupus was 'not active'. It took another six months and life being horrible with various symptoms, that I had to get angry and say I'd like someone to try and find out what was going on as they say the lupus wasn't active yet no one was willing to offer any help or advice as to what was wrong with me. I do not have a lupus nurse… didn't know they existed! And I see a rheumatologist every six months (for all it helps) and a kidney specialist (who is great, but can't deal with lupus symptoms, just the kidneys).

At present, for many of our respondents, the links we refer to above simply does not happen. People are often left to make sense of their own experiences, put the symptomatic two and two together and generate their own patchworks, the pieces of which mean little in isolation, like a jigsaw, they only create whole pictures when skilfully drawn together. We would suggest, therefore, that what appears to be missing from the clinical response to lupus, for some patients, is this coordination and connection role. This role would oversee and understand the multiplicities and complexities the condition presents to the person diagnosed and those charged with treating and supporting them and, in addition, would underscore the need to conceptualise bodies as genuinely whole, not clinically disaggregated entities.

   In the UK there are, in some specialist centres, lupus nurses (and nurses specialising in rheumatology more generally) who are able to chart a patient's journey through the lupus maze from diagnosis to treatment and long-term support, but this does require the patient to already exist on the lupus map. We would suggest that one of the professional groups very much absent in lupus is social work. As we will attest, none of the people we spoke to in the course of our work had seen, or considered seeing, a social worker, yet the profession is well-placed to enable people with lupus (and other difficult to negotiate conditions) to chart the difficult waters of their condition. Without the support noted above, for many of the people we spoke to in the course of this project, the lack of coordination, the seemingly random nature, not only of symptoms, but also the sometimes unsympathetic, unconnected and seemingly uninterested clinicians was a critical element in many unsatisfactory clinical encounters that, for some people, actually constituted an additional burden of illness – what might be referred to as iatrogenic clinical experiences (Illich, 1975).

> **Ann:** As new symptoms arise and become troublesome, you find yourself back *again* at the GP (who, incidentally, you feel must think you're some sort of hypochondriac) who scratches her head in bewilderment at another seemingly random set of complaints. Off you go for another round of tests that may or may not reveal something 'going on', but never do any of these people refer to your overarching condition and relate their own findings to it. It's as if your body is a range of completely unconnected parts that have nothing to do with each other. You begin to feel like a fraud and it feels as though you are somehow inappropriately taking up their time. When you go to visit the consultant, you worry about it for weeks on end, get really anxious and stressed (which does not help your condition!) and then, while some can be interested and engaged, you are often left feeling completely patronised and demeaned. It can leave you feeling really distressed and angry... to be honest, the temptation is just to get on with it yourself. I ask myself, what's the point of getting involved with the medics, because it just makes you feel worse.

What this quote illuminates is the 'contest' sometimes embodied in the clinical encounter in which the patient and physician are engaged in the same, yet clearly divergent, endeavours that are underpinned, as we have noted above, by a strongly practitioner-centred model 'in which the epistemological authority of medical knowledge and practice, paternalistically embodied in the doctor' is a given (May et al., 2004: 136).

In generating this critique, we are, of course, cognisant of the fact that, in this book, our concern is to capture and make sense of the experiences of people living with autoimmune conditions. An explication of the experiences and views of practitioners in this process, while clearly relevant, falls outside the remit of the text. It is therefore only the patients' experiences of the clinical encounter that we record here. While the literature on doctors' experiences of the clinical encounter is, itself rather sparse, Lupton (1997: 482) suggests that there is an extensive body of work which measures patient satisfaction with, and perceptions of, practitioners, ethnographies of medical work, studies of medical education and training and, of course, the hierarchical relationships between doctors and patients. Lupton (1997) and Nettleton et al. (2008) point out, however, that there is little sociological research that seeks to ascertain, 'practitioner satisfaction' and 'the emotional aspects of medical work'.

In their work on the 'emotional aspects of routine medical work', Watt et al. (2008) and Nettleton et al. (2008) point to the changing social and policy context that is significantly shaping the experience of medical practice (for patients and practitioners) in the early twenty-first century. In particular, they identify regulatory changes that have resulted in doctors witnessing 'a decrease in professional autonomy and increasing external accountability, monitoring and managerial controls' (Watt et al., 2008: 592). This is juxtaposed with a growing 'consumerist ethos' and widespread availability of medical knowledge, largely, as we have previously noted, because of the growth of online health sources and resources.[4] There are two findings from their research that pertain most immediately to our project. The first is the difficulties some doctors encountered when working in a context of clinical uncertainty. The second is the ambivalence that appeared to characterise a great deal of their practice. One such ambivalence is that of meeting the requirements of evidence-based practice, requiring rational, scientific, resource-led decision-making while balancing this with patient expectations that doctors, 'respect human dignity, be caring and express feelings such as empathy, sympathy and emotional sensitivity' (Watt et al., 2008: 596). As Nettleton et al. (2008: 34) argue: 'Ironically, at a time when doctors are being exhorted to adhere to evidence-based guidelines and protocols, and to eschew personalised and experiential knowledge (Harrison, 2002) they need greater "emotional intelligence" to negotiate with well-informed patients who have increasingly consumerist expectations.' It is, perhaps, the seemingly irreconcilable nature of these competing demands that may explain some of the ways in which these challenges are so evidently apparent to patients.

There is little doubt that the ideological shifts in care transition have recast the contemporary clinical encounter for both patients and practitioners. Expectations, roles, demands, requirements and responsibilities have altered in response to policy initiatives, service user/patient-led social movements and the clinical recognition of the value of joint medical working (between patients and professionals). However, our data also demonstrates the extraordinary tenacity of medical power and authority to resist these shifts and the unease that some patients demonstrate when asked to embrace their 'expert' status (in addition to clinicians' evident distrust of the concept). Thus, for our respondents, despite the changes noted above, the clinical encounter retains much of its traditional paternalistic and hierarchical form.

Lupus exposes some of the particular challenges embedded in the clinical encounter, particularly when facing and managing uncertainties given that autoimmune conditions, are themselves quintessentially uncertain in their diagnosis, prognosis and everyday lived reality. This condition demands very particular things from the clinical relationship, not least a recognition and acknowledgement of the nature and impact of uncertainty. Our data has suggested that this acceptance is particularly difficult to achieve. Moreover, lupus reveals the shortcomings of clinical encounters that are multiple and unconnected. Lupus, and its associated difficulties, highlights a range of particular clinical and interpersonal needs that, our data suggests, are not always effectively met or managed by all (and sometimes any) participants in the clinical relationship. This generates a potent combination that can come together to obfuscate and undermine the patient illness experience and it is to a further exploration of that day-to-day reality, therefore, that we now turn in Chapter 4.

## Notes

1  In using the term 'clinical encounter', we are referring broadly to the many occasions in which patients engage with health practitioners, although the data we draw on focuses specifically on patient interactions with consultants.

2 A collective term for a range of autoimmune diseases characterised by the presence of auto-antibodies (blood proteins), for example, lupus, scleroderma, Reynaud's syndrome.
3 See, for example, the Department of Health (2014) *2014/15 Choice Framework*.
4 See Chapter 6.

# References

Department of Health (1999) *Saving Our Lives: Our Healthier Nation*, www.gov.uk/government/uploads/system/uploads/attachment_data/file/265576/4386.pdf (accessed 17 November 2013).

Department of Health (2001) *The Expert Patient: A New Approach to Chronic Disease Management in the 21st Century*. London: The Stationery Office.

Department of Health (2004a) *Choosing Health: Making Healthy Choices Easier*, http://webarchive.nationalarchives.gov.uk/+/www.dh.gov.uk/en/Publicationsandstatistics/Publications/PublicationsPolicyAndGuidance/DH_4094550 (accessed 17 November 2013).

Department of Health (2004b) *The NHS Improvement Plan: Putting People at the Heart of Public Services*, http://webarchive.nationalarchives.gov.uk/+/www.dh.gov.uk/en/Publicationsandstatistics/Publications/PublicationsPolicyAndGuidance/DH_4084476 (accessed 17 November 2013).

Department of Health (2014) *2014/15 Choice Framework*, www.gov.uk/government/uploads/system/uploads/attachment_data/file/299609/2014-15_Choice_Framework.pdf (accessed 12 August 2014).

Gardner, J., Dew, K., Stubbe, M., Dowell, T. and Macdonald, L. (2011) 'Patchwork Diagnoses: The Production of Coherence, Uncertainty, and Manageable Bodies'. *Social Science & Medicine* 73: 843–850.

Giddens, A. (1991) *Modernity and Self Identity*. Cambridge: Polity Press.

Greenhalgh, T. (2009) 'Chronic Illness: Beyond the Expert Patient'. *British Medical Journal* 338(7695): 629–631.

Harrison, S. (2002) 'New Labour, Modernisation and the Medical Labour Process'. *Journal of Social Policy* 31: 465–485.

Illich, I. (1975) *Medical Nemesis: The Expropriation of Health*. New York: Pantheon Books.

Katz, J. (1987) Physician-Patient Encounters '*On a Darkling Plain*', http://digitalcommons.law.yale.edu/fss_papers (accessed 7 November 2013).

Laing, A., Newholme, T., Keeling, D., Speier, D., Hog, G., Minocha, S. and Davies, L. (2010) *Patients, Professionals and the Internet: Renegotiating the Healthcare Encounter*, www.nets.nihr.ac.uk/__data/assets/pdf_file/0006/64527/FR-08-1602-130.pdf (accessed 8 December 2013).

Lupton, D. (1997) 'Doctors on the Medical Profession'. *Sociology of Health and Illness* 19: 480–497.

May, C., Allison, G., Chapple, A., Chew-Graham, C., Dixon, C., Gask, L., Graham, R., Rogers, A. and Roland, M. (2004) 'Framing the Doctor–Patient Relationship in Chronic Illness: A Comparative Study of General Practitioners' Accounts'. *Sociology of Health & Illness* 26(2): 135–158.

Mol, A. (2002) *The Body Multiple: Ontology in Medical Practice*. Durham, NC, and London: Duke University Press.

Nettleton, S., Burrows, R. and Watt, I. (2008) 'How do You Feel Doctor? An Analysis of Emotional Aspects of Routine Professional Medical Work'. *Social Theory & Health* 6: 18–36.

NHS Executive (1998) *The New NHS Modern and Dependable: A National Framework for Assessing Performance*, www.qub.ac.uk/elearning/media/Media,259943,en.pdf (accessed 6 April 2014).

NHS Modernisation Agency (2004) *The Strategic Leadership of Clinical Governance in PCTs*, www.pilgrimprojects.co.uk/clients/nhsma/cg2/Section5.pdf (accessed 6 April 2014).

Novas, C., and Rose, N. (2000) 'Genetic Risk and the Birth of the Somatic Individual'. *Economy and Society* 29(4): 485–513.

Shaw, J. and Baker, M. (2004) 'Expert Patient – Dream or Nightmare?' *British Medical Journal* 328: 723–724.

Stockl, A. (2007) 'Complex Syndromes, Ambivalent Diagnosis, and Existential Uncertainty: The Case of Systemic Lupus Erythematosus (SLE)'. *Social Science & Medicine* 65: 1549–1559.

Taylor, D. and Bury, M. (2007) 'Chronic Illness, Expert Patients and Care Transition'. *Sociology of Health & Illness* 29(1): 27–45.

Thompson, C. J. (2003) 'Natural Health Discourses and the Therapeutic Production of Consumer Resistance'. *Sociological Quarterly* 44(1): 81–107.

Watt, I., Nettleton, S. and Burrows, R. (2008) 'The Views of Doctors on their Working Lives: A Qualitative Study'. *Journal of the Royal Society of Medicine* 101: 592–597.

Werner, A. and Malterud, K. (2003) 'It is Hard Work Behaving as a Credible Patient: Encounters Between Women with Chronic Pain and their Doctors'. *Social Science & Medicine* 57(8): 1409–1419.

Young, J. (2007) *The Vertigo of Late Modernity*. London: Sage.

# 4 A life lived with lupus

**Holly:** After having my third child last year I found things much more difficult. I found small tasks so hard. I presented at my doctor and the hospital several times with infections and pains. The doctor generally felt that my immune system was low after having the baby and I was just unlucky with infections. Also advised that breast-feeding reduces your immune [system]. I couldn't go on like this, I was really struggling.

I probably didn't really tell anyone how I was feeling, not now when I look back. I guess, as a mum, you have so much responsibility, especially with a newborn. You feel you have to cope, just keep going and surely you'll feel better soon.

On several occasions I experienced severe arthritic pains, which meant that I was unable to hold my baby, which was really tough, especially because I was breast-feeding. At the time, the doctor advised that I might have a reactive arthritis that flares when the body has infection. We discussed taking bloods to test me for arthritis. I decided to do this, as it was very severe at the time, although also completed vanished within a week or two… I also had mouth infections, as a result of lots of mouth ulcers. Again, the doctor was just of the view that my immune system was low and unable to fight infections on its own – the tiredness is the worst!

Anyway, I was given several courses of antibiotics; I would almost feel as though I was getting better when another infection would floor me. The hospital staff were good, but only treated my symptoms, no one ever queried previous infections or concerns.

I was at the doctors about four months ago and the nurse was taking bloods, I broke down, explained how I was feeling and how ill I felt. Quickly saw the doctor, who was very sympathetic and said you've got to tell us how you are feeling! Wish I done this sooner. Hindsight's great! Although I had been to the doctors lots, I was just telling him about a current infection at the time, I didn't know there was more going on. My partner was quite annoyed with the health service in general; he felt that they should have taken bloods a long time ago.

Anyway, blood results showed that my kidneys and lungs were not functioning properly, my blood pressure was also very high. I was admitted to hospital that day, I was actually relieved! Thinking that you can't cope or feel any worse… Least now, I knew why!

I stayed in hospital for almost one week, and my body recovered very well, with just rest. They took bloods three times every day and checked BP several times daily (initially catheterised). They just kept telling me things had improved and I was getting better. Kind of just relieved that I felt better again... until my discharge letter highlighted some concerns.

I was readmitted a couple of weeks later to do a kidney biopsy. The results show that it was my own body that attacked my kidneys, and they think that it may be lupus, I have been back several times and each time they take more bloods. Still querying it as lupus. I feel I need confirmation to allow acceptance and move on. When I was in hospital everyone was so worried and everyone emphasised that they were all there for me and very supportive, I didn't have to struggle through this alone! Everyone now is checking I'm alright, I'm really fortunate that way! But still find it emotionally very difficult... probably feel counselling would be beneficial, which I shall pursue when I'm finally diagnosed. I now have to change my lifestyle. I'm trying to be positive about this, but find it very difficult...

I think not having a diagnosis leaves me very unsettled. I was due to return to work last month, but feel I am not ready to do so. I would feel better if they knew what was wrong and advised what they can do to help. I worry how I'll cope returning to work.

Currently I find household tasks very tiring and don't cope very well if I don't get much sleep. I can be teary and tired and sore. The joys of parenthood and lupus!

I feel guilty too; I have to rely on others to help, with everyday tasks. I used to be so strong and independent.

I am very lucky that I have an amazing fiancé and a great daughter that helps me every day. Both grandparents are wonderful too! Overnights at granny's every week is a great break :-) I have considered asking my health visitor for support. I am unaware of support on the lupus website, but I shall have a nosy. In my job I tell people all the time to accept support before they are on their knees... now I understand (from the heart) how hard it really is to acknowledge that you can't manage on your own, whatever your age.

Anyway, I hope that my life can be as fulfilling as I planned, maybe just a bit more healthy, less alcohol, also planning my days and taking things very easy. Even though it's not in my nature, I know the benefits are far greater! Feeling well is bliss... I don't want to think too far ahead, my condition may not worsen, maybe that's very unrealistic, I'm not sure to be honest. I guess one step at a time.

It does worry me that I might not cope well at work and find this too stressful. I love my work! I didn't find it too stressful before, so hoping if I can reserve my energy, I'll manage just as well as I did before, although shall take things that little bit slower, if poss. Again, everyone in my work has been wonderful, so support-ive, especially my boss, it really, really helps! I tell myself that I shouldn't worry, 'cause I've got all their support right behind me.

My future plans shall have to be altered, maybe no more partying in the sun, instead just chilling in the shade – it could be worse.

Holly's story reflects many of the issues raised in the previous two chapters and also of many other people we spoke to. The range and seriousness of Holly's many symptoms gives some insight into the physiological complexity autoimmune conditions such as lupus present, while providing a simultaneous idea of how difficult they are to pinpoint and diagnose. In this context at least, Holly's story is far from unusual.

What her narrative also shapes is our understanding of what it is like to live with ongoing ill-health – the uncertainty and symptomatic ambiguity, the difficulties associated with naming the problem (diagnosis), the challenges autoimmune conditions such as lupus present for professionals and the impacts they can have in terms of a sense of self, one's personal and professional identity, the recalibration of future hopes and dreams and the importance of a reliable support system. Her story also points to the bewilderment engendered when it is patently one's body that is creating its own medical problems and, further, her narrative outlines the various ways in which ongoing illness fundamentally undermines the ways in which our bodies, and their relative well-being, symbolically denote our human value (Townsend, 2011).

In this chapter, we turn to an exploration of these issues – the lived experience of chronic illness, and of autoimmunity in particular. We are interested in how people understand and make sense of their illness and the ways in which it can impact on their day-to-day lives and experience. We explore, in particular, the meanings people attribute to illness and the ways in which they negotiate and manage it on a daily basis. We are interested to understand the ways in which autoimmunity can generate simultaneous destruction and possibility, transforming a life in the process. Indeed, it is often in the familiar, perhaps mundane practices of daily life that the most profound impacts of autoimmunity are evident. The taken-for-granted ordinariness of life is the very aspect that is most touched by these conditions, making them sometimes undetectable to the outside eye, yet nonetheless remarkable in their effects for those experiencing them.

## Finding a voice

The literature exploring lives lived with illness is extensive, but very much reflects the 'disciplinary sensibilities' (Thorne et al., 2002) of the various fields. Research from the applied health sciences, for example, tends to be grounded firmly in the practice perspective, focusing on methods of managing pain and alleviating suffering (Denny and Earle, 2009; Lloyd and Heller, 2012; Nicol, 2011) while that from psychology explores people's coping mechanisms and personal adaptations (Barlow, 2009; de Ridder et al., 2008) to the impacts of ill-health. Medical anthropologists, on the other hand, document patterns in beliefs about health and illness and locate them within wider social structures and cultural practices (Kleinmann, 1988, 2013; Stoller, 2004), while sociologists tend to be more interested in social and cultural rules and structures and the implications they have for people's understanding and behaviours in the context of ill-health. As such, the outcomes of research in this area are shaped by a disciplinary focus in terms of theoretical perspective, method and the manner in which findings are presented (Thorne et al., 2002). The ways in which people's illness experiences are reported and understood are reliant on a range of discreet yet interlinking factors, the researcher's disciplinary field being a case in point, although it is interesting to note that social work does not share the same tradition.

One way of obfuscating the researcher's disciplinary predilections (with a view to foregrounding the personal experience of illness) is to focus on personal narratives of illness, which allow for the individuation of experience that at once seems similar (in the context of symptoms and treatment approaches and outcomes) yet diverse, given that people may experience the same illness very differently. A dominant feature of the patient voice, and a space where narrative is most dominant, is, of course, biography and memoir (Carel, 2008; Conway, 2007; Edwards, 2013; Foster and Swander, 1998; Mairs, 1990). Illness narratives offer to uncover the 'truth' behind a person's experience, without being reflected or refracted through the researcher's disciplinary lens. They are at once a research tool and a naturalistic method people employ to try to make sense of their experience. It should be stressed, however, that it is rare to find narratives that stand alone without analysis or other reading. Exceptions would be *Voices of Scleroderma* (International Scleroderma Network, 2003) and the MS Project (Turner, 2011) in which patients' narratives are presented independently of external analysis. Here, we attempt to map something of a middle course through these traditions, quoting verbatim from respondents' accounts while providing our analysis of their narratives, thus maintaining our commitment to carefully foreground the voices of our respondents. In applied contexts, narrative work is a method of both research *and* intervention, as an exploration of the person's biography can help both them and the professionals working with them to make sense of their situation and to allow for wider connections to be made. In social work, in particular, the voice of the service user (in the context of our own work, the narrative of our respondents) is accorded a particular centrality.

The popularity of illness narratives is a relatively recent phenomenon which owes its upsurge to a number of academic and social contexts. Langellier (in Riessman, 2002: 2) suggests that this has arisen partially from the 'narrative turn' away from the positivist project in the social sciences; the rise in interest in the documentation of personal experience, what she refers to as the 'memoir boom'; the rise of 'identity movements' in which marginalised communities strive for emancipation, and an increasingly evident therapeutic culture – the exploration of personal life in therapies of various kinds. In turn, Riessman (2002: 3) suggests that illness narratives are a 'response to biomedicine's focus on disease, and consequent neglect of patients' embodied experience… [that] can provide a corrective to biomedicine's objectification of the body and, instead, embody a human subject with agency and voice' (Riessman, 2002: 4).

Techniques and methods that allow the person to make sense of their experience and, in so doing, to display and reflect that experience out toward the world, are powerful tools that enable them to more readily assimilate illness experiences into their sense of self and identity – something that illness may fundamentally undermine. It is, as we have variously outlined, when the unquestioned and taken for granted effective functioning of our bodies is destabilised, when our physical selves become ineffective and when our physical and existential interactions with the world become problematic, that we can begin to question our sense of self. 'Our body, in effect, moves us out into the world of social interactions and performances through which we come to constitute our sense of self' (Charmaz, 1991: 6). Physical illness that affects our personal, work, social and civil life undermines both our sense of self and, by definition, our place in the world. As we have already suggested, when that which causes the illness in the first place *is* one's own self, this process can be particularly profound. Meaning making, in this context, is not only necessary but perhaps even life-saving. 'Illness or, more accurately, our relationship to it, threatens the way we know ourselves and how others know us also. Anything that helps put illness in its place, that allows us to feel that we are who we are despite it, is welcome' (Weingarten, 2001).

Illness narratives, then, are ways in which people experiencing illness first-hand, and those around them, can make sense of, and give meaning to, their illness experience. As we stated in the introduction to this book, our own early experiences of ill-health were gradually woven into personal narratives that helped us each make sense of what initially seemed to be incomprehensible symptoms and equally incomprehensible and seemingly fruitless and exasperating encounters with professionals. Indeed, one of the ways we have each assimilated illness into our sense of self and identity is to employ our own familiar tools and approaches, resulting in research that focuses on the issues that, at first, seemed so oblique. We have used the insights gained to think and write about illness in an effort to make sense of our experiences. Other people's approaches would differ, no doubt, but this explanation of our own attempts at, and methods of, meaning-making perhaps underline our wider point.

Like any other account, however, first-person narratives are themselves inevitably mediated by a person's socio-cultural context, which the process of becoming and being ill simultaneously augments and undermines. 'Becoming chronically ill does not remove one from society; if anything it amplifies one's position in it, so that what people adjust *with* is as important a matter as what people attempt to adjust *to*' (Radley, 1989: 243). Thorne and Paterson (1998) provided an analysis of the changes to the ways in which the lives of people with chronic illness have been reported. They cite the most fundamental shift from exclusively outsider (largely biomedical) research methods to a more customary focus on the insider perspective and the various ways in which a variety of different lenses have been applied to the experience of chronic illness in this context. While notions of burden and loss characterised early work in the area, later studies have focused more explicitly on courage, hope, control, management and meanings of illness. 'The images collectively reveal an alternatively constructed orientation toward challenging the traditional loss and suffering focuses and uncovering those aspects of chronic illness that are healthy, transformative, and positive' (Thorne and Paterson, 1998: 175). While this turn of analytical events is clearly mediated upon an anti-oppressive obligation to focus more purposefully on the ill person's own perspective, there is, perhaps, a need to analyse the ways in which this tempers what is reported and how a person's experience is thus presented. While this development (the shift from a focus on burden and loss to the transformative effects of illness) clearly has advantages for people living with illness, i.e., that they are more often perceived as informed consumers who are partners and equal decision-makers in the context of their healthcare (although this, in itself, is questionable, in light of the experiences we related in Chapters 2 and 3) this approach might also serve to obfuscate the realities of living with illness in favour of a prerogative to purposefully foreground the transformative possibilities illness might present. Shifting the gaze to focus on the pursuit of wellness can serve to silence the public and private articulation of the embodied realities of living with illness, unless this articulation has the explicit purpose of highlighting its transformative and transcendental possibilities (Ehrenreich, 2009).

The mode of analysis, the researcher's disciplinary intentions and the ways in which illness experiences are personally and socially framed and reported can, thus, give critical shape to our understanding and, as research informs practice, practitioners, in an effort to undermine the loss/burden model of illness, should also be wary of losing sight of the physical realities of illness and their very real impact upon the person and their experience. In providing much-needed space for people to accurately articulate their experiences, it is equally important to recognise that subjective experiences of burden, loss, distress and disruption remain very real components of the corporeal experience of illness. In short, people's narratives must be read in the round. However uncomfortable the reading may be, focusing primarily on the transformative and positive aspects of illness (foregrounding notions of conquest and restitution) does not allow for an accurate articulation of the illness experience. However framed, of course, each person's account of their illness is equally valid, permitting the author to narrate their story in the way that is most resonant for them and we set out these various contexts here, merely to remind the reader that the 'truth' about illness experiences are personally, socially and politically contingent and can only be read as such.

## Framing the illness experience

Given that the advent of illness and the subsequent 'illness experience' are contingent on the condition, the person and their socio-cultural context, it is, of course, not possible to generalise, but there are a number of key themes, referred to by Charmaz (1991: 72) as a 'shared resonance', that are evident in many people's accounts of autoimmune conditions. They focus, in particular, on the processes by which people become ill, the onset of symptoms and the search for their meaning, the experience of treatment provided and the associated outcomes and prognosis. All reveal a shifting kaleidoscope that constitutes the lived experience of illness, which is conceptualised in a variety of ways. Most popularly, and perhaps most easily understood by those who do not experience chronic illness, is a linear trajectory model that denotes a phased process in which people follow a largely predictable path during which the person experiences symptoms, achieves a diagnosis and is then able to access treatment and either cure, long-term disability or death. In the context of chronic illness, and autoimmune conditions in particular, however, these standard models, while acknowledging the possibility of regressive and non-linear progression between the various steps (Paterson, 2001) are not necessarily helpful. There are, therefore, contrasting approaches to understanding the experience of chronic illness that more accurately elucidate and reflect the realities of living with an autoimmune condition.

Sanderson et al. (2011), for example, suggest a more nuanced explanatory model of the experience of illness that focuses on changing conceptions of a 'normal' life and, in the context of a life lived with illness – the normalisation of symptoms. Rather than illness being perceived simply as an end to 'normal life', Sanderson et al. (2011) suggest six 'shifting' normalities.

*Disrupted normality*, wherein symptoms are overwhelming and intrusive and there is a sense that normal life is not possible.

*Struggling for normality*, where people fight to maintain previous conceptions of normality, whatever the cost.

*Fluctuating normality*, when flares of disease activity are unpredictable and thus normal life comes and goes.

*Returning to normality*, when treatment is successful and the life previously anticipated is again a possibility.

*Continuing normality*, in which normal life continues unabated.

*Resetting normality*, whereby illness becomes part and parcel of everyday life – living with illness becomes 'the new normal'.

The ways in which illness intrudes on people's life experiences and the degrees to which people become immersed in the experience and management of illness are what most fundamentally underpin any explanatory or exploratory model of chronic illness. Miles (2013: 12) provides a stark illustration of this in her study of Ecuadorian women with lupus:

> For some, lupus is a disruption in their life trajectory that sidetracked but did not derail them. These women occasionally feel tired, stiff, and sore, and they responded by monitoring their diets, medication, and stress levels. But for others, lupus, and caring for lupus, has become the central and dominating motif of daily life as a life threatening flare always seems to looming, even simple activities are often too much, and they found themselves constantly in and out of doctors' offices and hospitals in an attempt to control symptoms.

Charmaz (1991) offers a three point conceptual schema for understanding the ways in which illness is assumed into a person's life. She refers to each discreet yet critically interlinked point as interruption and intrusion by, and immersion in, illness. People may shift between states in what might be unpredictable 'bumps and jolts and long smooth stretches' (Charmaz, 1991: 9) and the particular point a person finds themselves at will determine the degree to which illness is foregrounded in their lives. Each person's initial experience of their illness will also, from this perspective, be different in that, for some, illness is a stealthy companion that slowly comes into focus, while, for others, acute illness is the herald of a more long-term condition that, from the beginning, is very much in the foreground of daily life. It is the person's own definitions of themselves and their illness that determine where in this triumvirate of experience they position themselves and are, by definition, placed.

Frank (1995), similarly, offers a model for understanding the experience of illness employing a description of three narrative styles; restitution, chaos and quest narratives. The restitution narrative involves a person, after a period of illness, returning to their previous, pre-illness self. Illness, in this context, is an interruption to normal life. The individual's responsibility, in this context, is to get well, the professional's responsibility is to enable recovery. The chaos narrative, as the term suggests, focuses more explicitly on a lack of control and meaning in illness, with the ill person lacking the agency so visibly apparent in the restitution narrative. The quest narrative, on the other hand, centres upon illness as an opportunity for transformation and transcendence – a spiritual journey.

A person's experience of illness might, however, reflect one or perhaps all narrative strands at different points, but what is clear from these various articulations, and was evident in the narratives of many of our respondents, is that linearity, in the context of autoimmunity – the smooth movement from symptom, to diagnosis, to prognosis and outcome – is not possible. In this context, Paterson (2001) suggested a 'shifting perspectives' model. She rejects linear models of illness trajectory in favour of a model that allows for the foregrounding of *either* illness or wellness at any point in the illness experience. As such, the illness 'journey' need not have an identified end (or indeed beginning) point and would not rely upon progression through easily identified stages before a certain point can be reached. Rather, it is a model that allows for a complex interaction and articulation between a person's self and their world (Paterson, 2001: 23).

Paterson's model is of particular interest to us, as the two variant perspectives (illness in the foreground or wellness in the foreground) offered contrast profoundly, the first focusing on the sickness, suffering and the various losses associated with living with long-term ill-health and the second, the wellness in the foreground perspective, privileging illness as an opportunity for meaningful change in a person's relationships and environment. The two facets of the model effectively underpin the two types of illness narrative we highlighted earlier – the deficit approach and the stoicism in the face of adversity model.

These various models could well be applied to our respondents' narratives in which a range of critical themes came together to allow a composite picture to develop from the often fragmentary patchwork of illness experiences they presented. The question remains, of course, whether it is actually possible to provide an explanatory framework for the lived experience of autoimmunity where the paradox of living with an illness in which the self attacks the self remains, we would argue, irresolvable. Despite the daily challenges that our respondents face and the inevitable question the autoimmune paradox generates – 'Do I hate myself?', people still need to find coherence and make sense of lives that are lived, not necessarily in the shadow of illness, but have a constant, though shifting, presence in the village of the sick (Stoller, 2004).

## Creating coherence from the incomprehensible: life with lupus

We have already focused on symptoms and the early experience of lupus in Chapters 2 and 3, where we outlined people's experiences of the onset of symptoms

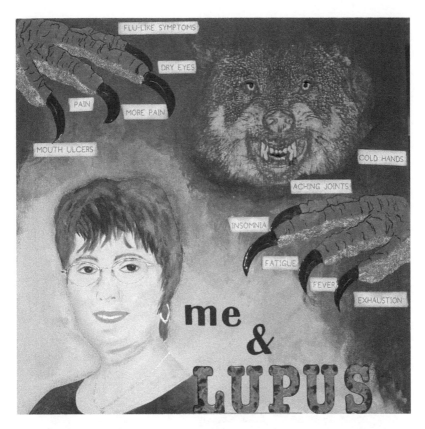

*Figure 4.1 Me and Lupus.* Reproduced with kind permission from the artist, Carole Chisholm.

and the diagnostic process. Here, we want to continue to follow people's journeys through the experience of autoimmunity to highlight, in particular, the day-to-day experience of living with an autoimmune condition. People have always chosen to represent and make sense of the experience of illness through a range of mediums and, as part of our lupus project, we wanted to focus beyond the spoken word. We asked our respondents if they would be willing to draw their illness in order to provide an alternative mode of expression for issues and feelings which can be so hard to articulate. The work of Padfield (2003), who explores the experience of pain and its expression and use in the clinical encounter, is of particular note in this context. Her work empowers patients to make visual (and visceral) the extent and effects of their pain through the use of photographic images. We were astounded by some of the work that resulted from our request and wanted to reproduce it here to provide an alternative reading of the experience of living with lupus. This work focuses, in particular, on the pain and disruptions living with an autoimmune condition can generate, but also highlights the ways in which illness and its management can present perhaps unimagined or anticipated opportunities for growth and

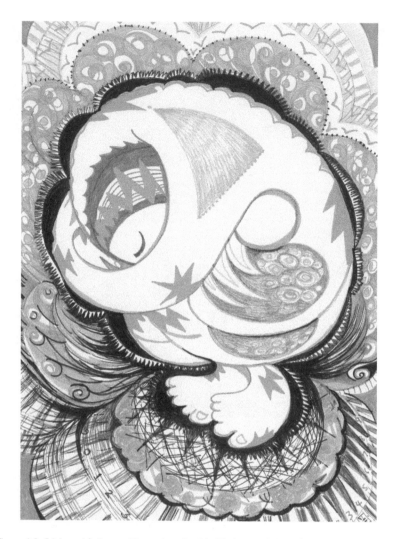

*Figure 4.2 Living with Lupus.* Reproduced with kind permission from the artist, Lin-Marie Milner Brown.

personal reflection that can have a positive benefit to the person who is ill and those who support them.

A key issue, as we have said many times, is the unpredictability of autoimmune symptoms and the varied professional responses to them. Illness, as we have outlined, is something that, in popular understanding, comes and then, with the correct treatment and support, goes again – a person is 'cured' and can return to their previous life. With autoimmune conditions, this is often not the case, as there are enduring issues to manage and maintain. Their unpredictability makes the distinction between acute and chronic illness particularly difficult to determine, as a person may seem quite well one day and acutely ill the next (reflecting, perhaps, Sanderson's et al.'s (2011) notion of shifting normalities and Paterson's (2001) foregrounding model) – these conditions do not follow a predictable script. Many people in our study expressed a sense of confusion and helplessness in the face of symptoms that shifted in and out of focus sometimes on a daily, or even hourly, basis.

> **Kerry:** Yeah, because I don't know what lupus is, I don't know what is going to happen from day to day, I don't know how it's going to attack me from one minute to the other I suppose.

> **Gina:** Some days I'd go in [to work] and I'd be fine, you know, have a really good day, but you couldn't get your head round the fact the next day I could be the complete opposite… My friend's coming with me [on holiday], you know, just to make it a little bit easier, because I could get up on that day and I won't be able to lift a case or a bag, I can't even bear my handbag on my shoulder, nothing, or I could get up and I'll be fine, and it's that not knowing.

This unpredictability had consequences for the people with lupus and their families and friends who also lived the roller-coaster of not knowing, day to day, if a person would be able to fulfil obligations and carry out planned work and activities. Even the possibility of becoming ill can serve as a barrier for both people with lupus and their friends and family. Ongoing and unpredictable ill-health undermines plans, routines and the continuity of daily life (Barker, 2005). It is the unpredictability and the not knowing if one will be well or ill on a particular day that can be such a frustrating feature of lupus and is a feature of other autoimmune diseases such as MS, RA and scleroderma. Flares of disease activity can happen at any time and people are required to be particularly vigilant regarding their own illness triggers (which may be different for each person). Charmaz (1991: 5) comments upon the way in which a disease flare effectively undermines a person's capacity to maintain routines and the continuity of daily life. 'A "good" day permits an even schedule and is savoured. A "bad" day forces attending to immediate needs and may be dreaded. Good days and bad days lends new meanings to the present and future and shade memories of the past.' As such, illness can be circumnavigated or become all-consuming depending upon its vagaries at any point.

This all-consuming feature is referred to by Charmaz (1991: 76) as an 'immersion in illness', wherein illness is no longer simply an unwelcome intrusion into life but, by necessity, life itself becomes founded on the experience of illness. She states 'no longer can people add illness to the structure of their lives; instead, they must *reconstruct* their lives upon illness. Illness, therefore, comes to shape a person's life and effectively define who they are and what they can do – their life is founded upon illness' (Charmaz, 1991) and their 'self' is reconstituted in the shadow of their condition. Charmaz makes a distinction, however, between a life founded upon illness and immersion in illness, the critical boundary between the two states being flares of disease activity. Here we can also refer back to the work of Paterson (2001) and the model of illness that situates illness either in the foreground or background. While illness is a constant feature of life, a variety of issues can exacerbate slippage and a shift into the illness in the foreground and the immersion context – this may be a flare of disease activity or a life event. Either way, with an autoimmune condition, a person's grasp of a sense of physical and emotional well-being is often tenuous and fleeting. Everyday activities must be reshaped in the shade cast by illness. Family, work and social life are all altered by illness and its consequences and, whether illness is foregrounded or is a more distant companion, there are inevitable effects on a person's sense of identity and self-worth. For our respondents with lupus, nowhere was this more evident than in the context of work and employment.

## The functional economy and the world of work

Illness variously impacts upon people's ability to undertake paid employment and an employer's response to illness is a critical factor in determining whether or not it is possible to continue to work. Again, the unpredictability of lupus symptoms and the fatigue that accompanies lupus made maintaining employment particularly difficult, especially for those who had physically demanding jobs.

> **Gina:** At work, I'd like sneak off and sit, put the lid down on the toilet and just… And have a little sit and put my head to one side and just sleep and it was awful and then, you know, all this anxiety and fear of, oh my God, if I fell asleep and didn't wake up and the embarrassment of it and, you know, you, you just can't continually be telling people all the time, you're tired, you're tired.

Work and the impact of illness on people's careers and future plans in this context were a common feature of their narratives, as they struggled to come to terms with altered futures and changes in, or, for some people, the ending of careers (as outlined in Amanda's experience p. 41).

A coherent sense of self and identity is inevitably affected by problems in the workplace and, clearly, by employers who may fail to grasp some of the realities of living with lupus. Indeed, the lack of support at work was a common feature of people's stories and, perhaps, a further measure of the lack of social meaning given to symptoms that are variable and often vague in character.

> **Ellie:** I loved my job and, like most in the job, social work was a major part of my life. But I was off sick a lot and this affected how I was treated… the 'caring' professions are not so caring when someone has a long-term illness! After many years of being told I was 'neurotic' I was finally diagnosed with a milder form of lupus – although if this is the affect mild disease has, my heart goes out to those with serious complications. I have had to retire on ill-health grounds as I can no longer commit to certain days/hours of work.

Many people gave up work (either by necessity or voluntarily) when they realised the effect it had on their health and the ways in which illness undermined their ability to carry out the tasks they had been employed to do.

**Gina:** I reduced all my hours at work, I couldn't work a full day anymore, I was only working until lunch-time, coming home just sleeping through the afternoon, one day just like was going into another day so of course that was making me anxious because… I've always been a very hyper sort of person, very hyperactive, doing ten things at once, you know, stressful jobs… it was always go, go, go for me, and then all of a sudden I was feeling, but I can't do anything… eventually went back to work but I wasn't coping. Okay, the pain had lessened, but I was actually, I was quite restricted in a lot of things I could do, I was still going to work and just those few hours, half a day, was exhausting so whatever energy I had went totally in going into work and then after that I was good for nothing, I literally had to just sleep until the next day when I got up again.

What was also evident in people's stories about illness and employment was a palpable sense of loss of both the direct financial benefits of being employed and a perhaps less tangible sense of the ways in which these various losses impact upon a person's sense of self and, in an effort to maximise functionality in the workplace, some people found their lives became shrunken to a work, eat and sleep regime with little room for anything else.

These issues highlight what might be termed (after Barker, 2005) the functional economy of lupus. Popularly known, particularly in the online environment, as 'spoon theory' (Miserandino, no date), which serves to conceptualise the ways in which a person marries up the limited amounts of energy they have at their disposal and the various tasks to be undertaken in any one day. In the context of fibromyalgia, Barker (2005) outlines the various strategies people use to manage restriction and the new and often limited parameters that life with chronic illness entails. She refers to the boundaries of a life founded upon illness that gradually (or, for some people, in a more acute manner) become determinants of a life strategy – one of restriction, reduction and the management of limited existential and physical ability.

The physical and psychological boundaries constituting what is possible on a day-to-day basis are often difficult to maintain and the transgression of these boundaries often results in further pain, suffering and distress. In this context, time, activities and suffering are closely monitored, assessed and variously managed. Given the limited physiological and psychological resources people have at their disposal, transgressions of their personal boundaries can become increasingly frequent as the illness takes its toll, with the concomitant shrinking of possibility. Referring to this process in economic terms is particularly apt, as both Ware (1999) and Barker (2005) refer to the need to 'bank' energy, to 'pay back' for over exertion or enthusiasm and to 'pay the price' for knowingly transgressing the limitations of energy. As such, when an illness is unpredictable, the available parameters for the management of restriction and the boundaries that contain a person's energy levels become increasingly inflexible.

**Corrine:** I think we do have control over our bodies, but when you are going through the transition to illness it takes time to get to grips with it. Prior to being ill, I'd say I knew my body well, having been very fit, and could push my body without any real consequences, other than the odd injury. Now, though, I have to try to coax my body to do things, and make sure that when I take exercise, for example, very carefully. I'm learning to tune into a different body in so many ways. With lupus, I am learning that it is important to not push myself too far, as it can lead to a return of symptoms, even if this isn't a 'flare'.

**Meg:** I have got to stick to the routine of going to bed at 9pm and if I go to bed later I will be trying to catch up all week without the right amount of rest, and measuring the amount of effort I put into each day I have been able to keep myself well in not having continual coughs and colds etc. Others around me have a hard time understanding that if I don't sleep at 9pm at night I will not be able to work the following day. Friends and workmates can be like 'it is only one night, go on', but I will pay for it at some point.

As lupus can flare up for no apparent reason, it is difficult, if not sometimes impossible, to predict or manage the course of the condition, the ways in which one's activities might impact upon it and vice versa. Laura highlights the impact this has had upon her life and the far reaching personal repercussions her condition generates.

**Laura:** I have fewer friends now than I did – I used to be very sociable and out every weekend and meeting friends during the week. But now I just don't have the energy. By the time the weekend comes around I'm so tired from work that I need to relax and recharge my batteries for the following week.

A lot of my friends live in different cities to me now and I don't have the energy to go and visit them so I've lost touch with a lot of them. A lot of my friends live abroad as well, so I keep in contact with them via e-mail, which is much easier for me.

Some of my older friends don't understand how much I have to pace myself now and so we've lost touch. They're the ones I think of as 'good times' friends. My 'true' friends stick by me.

As people experience and manage the restrictions and limitations imposed on their lives by lupus, they come to re-evaluate and reconstruct themselves in the context of their ongoing ill-health. That is, – they discover "the meaning of their altered bodies" (Charmaz, 1991: 21) and, for many people, their sense of self was fundamentally changed by lupus, as the limitations on their previous work, family and social worlds became increasingly foregrounded. Indeed, the ongoing construction of 'self', which we have referred to elsewhere and which we all engage in day-to-day, is fundamentally undermined by autoimmunity. Most critically, our physical body is our essential two-way conduit from and to the world and the undermining of that integrity by autoimmunity constitutes what Kleinmann (1988) refers to as a breach of the fundamental trust we implicitly place in our physical selves. As we alluded to in Chapter 1, the supposed unproblematic relationship between ourselves and our bodies and the ways in which it is undermined by autoimmunity, forces, for some, a critical re-evaluation of identity and self concept, while simultaneously impelling a re-evaluation of people's futures in light of an altered present (Charmaz, 1991; Gordon and Benishek, 1996; Gordon et al., 1998). It is to these issues that we turn in the following chapter.

# References

Barker, K. K. (2005) *The Fibromyalgia Story: Medical Authority and Women's Worlds of Pain*. Philadelphia: Temple University Press.

Barlow, J. (2009) *Living with Arthritis*. Oxford: BPS Blackwell.

Carel, H. (2008) *Illness: The Art of Living*. Durham: Acumen Publishing Limited.

Charmaz, K. (1991) *Good Days, Bad Days*. New Brunswick: Rutgers University Press.

Conway, K. (2007) *Ordinary Life: A Memoir of Illness*. Ann Arbor: University of Michigan Press.

Denny, E. and Earle, S. (2009) *Sociology for Nurses*. Cambridge: Polity.

de Ridder, D., Genen, R., Kuijer, R. and van Middendorp, H. (2008) 'Psychological Adjustment to Chronic Disease'. *Lancet* 372: 246–255.

Edwards, L. (2013) *In the Kingdom of the Sick: A Social History of Chronic Illness in America*. New York: Walker Publishing Company.

Ehrenreich, B. (2009) *Smile or Die: How Positive Thinking Fooled America and the World*. London: Granta Pulbications.

Foster, P. and Swander, M. (eds) (1998) *The Healing Circle: Authors Writing of Recovery*. New York: Plume.

Frank, A. (1995) *The Wounded Storyteller*. Chicago: University of Chicago Press.

Gordon, P. A. and Benishek, L. A. (1996) 'The Experience of Chronic illness: Issues of Loss and Adjustment'. *Journal of Personal and Interpersonal Loss* 1(3): 299–307.

Gordon, P. A., Feldman, D. and Crose, R. (1998) 'The Meaning of Disability: How Women with Chronic Illness View Their Experience.' *Journal of Rehabilitation* 64(3): 5–11.

International Scleroderma Network (2003) *Voices of Scleroderma*. Boston: International Scleroderma Network.

Kleinmann, A. (1988) *The Illness Narratives: Suffering, Healing & the Human Condition*. New York: Basic Books.

Lloyd, C. E. and Heller, T. (2012) *Long Term Conditions: Challenges in Health and Social Care*. London: Sage Publications Ltd.

Mairs, N. (1990) *Carnal Acts*. New York: HarperCollins.

Miles, A. (2013) *Living with Lupus: Women and Chronic Illness in Ecuador*. Austin: University of Texas Press.

Miserandino, C. (no date) *The Spoon Theory*, www.butyoudontlooksick.com/articles/written-by-christine/the-spoon-theory (accessed 9 April 2015).

Nicol, J. (2011) *Nursing Adults with Long Term Conditions*. London: Sage.

Padfield, D. (2003) *Perceptions of Pain*. Stockport: Dewi Lewis Publishing.

Paterson, B. L. (2001) 'The Shifting Perspectives Model of Chronic Illness'. *Journal of Nursing Scholarship* 33(1): 21–26.

Radley, A. (1989) 'Style, discourse and constraint in adjustment to chronic illness'. *Sociology of Health & Illness*. 11(3) 230–252.

Riessman, C. K. (2002) *Illness Narratives: Positioned Identities*, www.cardiff.ac.uk/encap/resources/HCRC-narratives.pdf (accessed 25 October 2013).

Sanderson, T., Calnan, M., Morris, M., Richards, P. and Hewlett, S. (2011) 'Shifting Normalities: Interactions of Changing Conceptions of a Normal Life and the Normalisation of Symptoms in Rheumatoid Arthritis', *Sociology of Health & Illness* 33(4): 618–633.

Stoller, P. (2004) *Stranger in the Village of the Sick: A Memoir of Cancer, Sorcery and Healing*. Boston: Beacon Press.

Thorne, S. and Paterson, B. (1998) 'Shifting Images of Chronic Illness'. *Journal of Nursing Scholarship* 30(2): 173–178.

Thorne, S., Paterson, B., Acorn, S., Canam, C., Joachim, G. and Jilling, C. (2002) 'Chronic Illness Experience: Insights from a Metastudy'. *Qualitative Health Research* 12(4): 437–452.

Townsend, A. (2011) 'Working to Manage Chronic Illness in Daily Life'. *Occupational Therapy Now* 13(5): 20–22.

Turner, L. (2011) *The MS Project: Orange is the New Pink* (Volume I), www.lainaturner.com/book-category/the-ms-project-series (accessed 2 May 2014).

Ware, N. C. (1999) 'Toward a Model of Social Course in Chronic Illness: The Example of Chronic Fatigue Syndrome'. *Culture, Medicine and Psychiatry* 23: 303–331.

Weingarten, K. (2001) *Making Sense of Illness Narratives*, www.dulwichcentre.com.au/illness-narratives.html (accessed 8 October 2013).

# 5 Foreclosed futures and lost pasts

## Reconstituting a salvaged self [1]

**Ola:** I was a 38-year-old mum, slim and very fit when I suddenly developed lupus on holiday in Malaysia, along with a severe dose of traveller's tummy. But looking back, I'm not surprised that I developed a disease where my body attacks itself. Throughout my childhood I suffered extensive abuse at home and at school. My mum didn't want a girl and throughout her life she continued to tell me I should never have been born and that having me had ruined her life. So I was physically fit, but mentally destroyed inside, with very low self-esteem and constantly under verbal attack within my family. Hardly surprising then that my immune system eventually joined in the attack.

At first lupus took over my life somewhat because it was uncontrolled, but I continued to play sports and do everything else as much as normal as possible, given some days my joints were so swollen I could hardly move and my speech, memory and balance were affected and I was having absences. I was determined from the start that lupus wasn't going to beat me.

Once I was put on azathioprine life improved no end. I still have regular flare ups and the fatigue can be very depressing at times, but I've stuck to my decision not to let lupus be my identity or run my life. Most people who know me at work have no idea that I have lupus, they know me for who I am and what I do.

Over the last three years I've had surgery a number of times for skin cancers, caused the doctors think by long-term azathioprine use. Cancers on my face have challenged my identity, as did losing part of my eye to cancer, but whenever I've withdrawn from azathioprine, lupus has returned with a vengeance. Plastic surgeons are wonderful and my face looks fine now more or less.

What's helped me keep an identity separate from lupus has been becoming a Christian three years ago in the midst of cancer surgery – a wonderful nurse offered to pray for me and the healing that followed amazed the doctors. Now I know that whatever I look like outwardly and whatever lupus does, I am accepted in God's eyes and loved and my Christian friends love me and respect me for who I am.

This year lupus has been causing psychosis when it flares up and that's been very scary. That's something I still have to get to grips with and with the help of a very caring psychiatrist and mental health nurse I'm sure we'll work out how best to manage the psychosis, but it hasn't changed who I see myself as and no one sees me as 'mad'.

My husband, now grown-up kids and my friends have been brilliant and life continues as usual, with the odd short break while I take time out now and then during a lupus flare with a psychotic episode.

I trust to God to get me through this difficult time, like all the other difficulties in life, and He never lets me down. I'm fortunate to have friends praying for me too and they still love me and I can still work part-time and still go out on the streets to help the homeless and do other outreach work that I enjoy. Life is good because I'm now loved and accepted for who I am and it doesn't matter if I have lupus or anything else.

For Ola, illness and its effects are assimilated and managed, her identity, she insists, exists separately to her illness, which is compartmentalised and resisted – her sense of self remains intact and life's valued roles and responsibilities remain at the forefront of experience despite the extraordinary way in which her words speak to the nature of the autoimmune paradox – 'looking back, I'm not surprised that I developed a disease where my body attacks itself'. Her narrative, it seems, very much reflects a life in the present but, for many of our respondents, it was the anticipated (and often very much feared future) that often dominated a narrative.

As we have noted in the previous chapter, lupus, like many incurable conditions, imposes the necessity to re-evaluate a sense of self, which is, for many people, diminished by their condition. One's identity is challenged and called into question by a disease process that undermines both the biological and existential relationship ordinarily enacted in the world around us. In this process, the passage of time garners increasing significance, as the anticipated future (the one planned and hoped for) is unlikely to fully materialise.

This chapter follows closely from the last, in that we again foreground the narratives of our respondents as they journey through the everyday, often mundane, corporeal realities of living with illness. Here, as the quote above starkly illustrates, we focus on the autoimmune imperative to renegotiate the self or, at very least, 'to reinstate the normal condition of self tolerance' (Anderson and Mackay, 2014). The focus of this chapter, however, is very much on how the illness journey informs and impacts upon the future and how people make sense of their futures in light of their shifting and uncertain present.

## Illness and the changing self

While Ola strongly asserted that her identity should remain separate from her diagnosis, there was, for many of our respondents, a sense that an ill self constituted a quite new self, one that was neither sought, nor necessarily welcomed. While illness, therefore, is the progenitor of that new self, it also, paradoxically, constitutes a central defining feature of the newly constituted self. The process by which this occurs, in other words, the ways in which people have sought to reconstitute themselves (in spite of 'themselves') is another central and paradoxical feature of the autoimmune experience. This new self demands a resetting of life's priorities and a profound re-evaluation of what it means to be 'me', particularly where 'me' has the same essential identity as the 'me' that is causing the disruption in the first place. What we identified in our data was a sense that people were engaged in this process at different points at different times (again, not necessarily a linear process), but that the undermining of self and its gradual reconstitution in the context of living with an autoimmune condition, was existential work that everyone was purposefully engaged in.

Some people invoked a sense of loss of self (without sight of any subsequent re-emergence). The destructive (autoimmune) self has, indeed, foreclosed the future and also, for some, the present. Ellie underlines this point particularly well, invoking the notion of becoming an invisible 'non-person', illness having stripped away a sense of her pre-illness identity. Loving, yet having a sense of being unlovable, physically changed by the illness and its treatment and only able to look forward to the next, eagerly anticipated, period of relative well-being.

> **Ellie:** I am fortunate and do work from home flexibly to suit myself, tutoring – however, it isn't really where my heart is! I feel a 'non-person' now, with little identity, even less social life and altogether invisible really. That sounds negative and I guess I feel that way presently – as most people do in the midst of a flare, which I am having right now. I have two great grown sons, due to be a gran next year and I should be delirious. Instead, I am eager not to burden my sons with my misery although they are on the whole very understanding having grown up with me like this.
>
> I have little self-esteem (It was never in short supply when well!) and my body image is appalling even more so that I have given up smoking and had to have intermittent steroids, all of which add to my bulk, which has never been slim! I want to be loved like anyone else, but feel that no one would understand my inability to be full of energy most of the time – and anyway it is hard to meet men when you need to plan for weeks for a night out in order to have the rest needed.
>
> I know I sound a moaning minnie, and really I know there are many others who suffer with this horrid illness much more than myself, but it is the emotional consequences of this (and other) chronic illness that are the worst to bear, the lack of identity, isolation and loneliness that come with it. Roll on remission, that's what I say...

In a bid to begin to make sense of this experience, many people felt a need to compare their pre-illness selves to the changed ill person they had become. Corrine, in juxtaposing her pre- and actively ill self, provides a particularly stark example of this contrast.

> **Corrine:** SLE like other chronic illnesses, I believe, can strip the heart right out of you and change you into something that you don't recognise in the mirror anymore. Yes, after four years of being diagnosed I'm still in mourning for the 'girl' I once was...

Adjectives I'd use to describe me:

| PAST | PRESENT |
| --- | --- |
| Slim | Very fat |
| Attractive | Unattractive |
| Sexy | Frump |
| Mentally quick | Mentally slow |
| Funny | A bit depressing |
| Sociable | Unsociable |
| Successful | Failure |
| Energetic | Tired |
| Motivated | Unmotivated |
| Proud of myself | Ashamed |
| In control | Not in control |
| Content | Okay |
| No guilt | Guilty |
| Liked pressure | Hate pressure |
| A somebody | A nobody |

Failure, ashamed and guilty are biggies for me – I'm separated because my husband didn't understand the illness so wasn't supportive at all (I asked him to leave as part of my de-stress your life campaign) = failed marriage. I haven't managed to overcome my illness, remain positive and return to work – I'm not a martyr, but a failure.

I'm on incapacity benefit and don't foresee a return to any form of career that includes pressure/stress or quick thinking and I'm on the list for a council property. I'm obese and my son has just started saying that he doesn't want a 'fat' mummy anymore = ashamed (have started a diet AGAIN!).

I have two fairly young children who have suffered more than me really due to the separation and the fact that mummy doesn't have the energy or isn't physically capable to do everything they/I would like to do. And I can't provide for them very well financially anymore = guilty.

Socialising is a BIG effort, not only do I worry about what to wear to try to cover my bulges but also what to say. I avoid social interaction with people who I don't know well because I hate sounding like an idiot when I word search or say the wrong word or am just slow. My memory has been affected and it takes time for me to retrieve the info. I'd like to wear a badge saying 'I'm not stupid, I'm ill' but that may seem like I'm attention-seeking rather than just stating a fact – we Brits should still just grin and bear it don't you know!

I don't know who I am anymore as an individual, but I do know that being a mum is the only thing that is keeping me going otherwise I'd just eat, sleep, read and watch TV.

I am always trying to work out how to manage life in the context of the illness! Not fantastically well is probably the answer, I find it difficult not to blame myself, not to think that I can make it better by working harder and pushing myself. I find it very difficult to be nice to myself and forgiving when I feel unwell. I miss the person that I was before the illness, and feel that I must be in some way responsible for the illness. When I have periods of being better I always believe that it will stay that way and find it devastating when things are worse. Basically coming to terms with the illness is very difficult, that said I guess I do manage, my stubbornness is a double-edged sword that keeps me going, but stops me from accepting the illness!

The loss of a sense of identity in a range of contexts is palpable in these words. Corrine's narrative is replete with guilt, regret and shame. Her sense of self is lost in the miasma of illness and her identity in those same contexts overshadowed by a profound sense of failure. Not managing to come to terms with her condition, and return to the pre-illness state, is perceived as further evidence of failure. This, of course, is made particularly acute when read in the context of autoimmunity, as the illness itself is an evident failure *of* the self.

For others, the process of reconstituting the self consisted of a need to critically re-evaluate each aspect of life in light of, and with evident deference to, lupus. In this context, lupus becomes an, undoubtedly unwelcome, life companion.

Amanda, for example, actually states that she became someone different:

My entire life plan had come to an end and I felt that I was useless, worthless, ugly and a failure and that I was a burden to everyone. I was ashamed and didn't want anyone who had known me before to see what I had become.

I had to go through a bereavement process, grieving for my old self… It was long, tough and arduous.

The first light at the end of the tunnel was going to university, as I was achieving something positive, albeit a struggle. I also met new friends who liked me as I was and would come to me for advice or emotional support as they noticed I had a caring nature. My course faculty have also been amazingly supportive.

As I got stronger emotionally and my lupus became more controlled, I have been able to increase my mobility, start exercising, lose some weight and have seen the old person re-emerge, although wiser and slightly different. I realised that my lifestyle could be adapted to help manage my lupus and again, this proactive approach helped renew my sense of self.

Three years post-diagnosis, I have my sense of self and identity back and have adapted my lifestyle and future goals to include managing my lupus.

Lupus is part of me but not all of me and this experience has taught me valuable lessons.

My new life is different to my old one and I actually prefer it now; I am quieter, calmer and more spiritual. I know myself well and have an inner peace. I no longer crave my old job but see myself taking my experience as a nurse and a patient with me into a future where I can care for people in an emotional rather than physical way.

For Amanda, her sense of self was gradually redefined and reconstituted through a new set of social and family relations. 'Self' was lost, but gradually reclaimed from the partiality of illness.

While some people in our study clearly would not or could not attain or seek this sense of resolution with their condition, others did see their experience as an opportunity for personal transformation and a fundamental reshaping of their life-world. Charmaz (1991) refers to this continuum as the range from loss to transcendence. The losses associated with living with autoimmune conditions are easily read in the narratives we have highlighted here; the possibilities for growth and transcendence are, perhaps, much more obliquely evident. Charmaz (1991: 257), in particular, focuses on the ways in which cumulative loss can result in a loss of self, that is, 'being involuntarily dispossessed of former attributes and sentiments that comprise one's self concept, as well as the actions and experiences upon which they are based'.

> **Gina:** And the illness made me give up my work, which was the last little bit of independence I had, I lost the house, I'd lost the husband, and then losing the job, you know.

As we noted above, in the face of illness, previous self concepts shift and change as illness impacts upon everyday experience and a person's self-concept can become vulnerable and increasingly permeable to the outside world. Again, this reflects a fundamental irony in the experience of autoimmunity, given that, as human beings, it is the outside world that we are, at least biologically, predisposed to resist. The paradox is further underlined given that, while it *may* be possible to resist the 'outside', it is, as these conditions so clearly illustrate, sometimes not possible to resist ourselves. The self, fundamentally at odds with the self, is engaged in a battle to at once overcome and then reconstitute itself.

Transcendence of this state implies acceptance of the illness and its meanings, it forces a re-evaluation of life and its purpose and an active approach to renewal and change. Both sides of this existential coin arise from both the experience of illness and the meanings people imbue it with (Charmaz, 1991). Charmaz is careful to point out that these two oppositional states are not necessarily mutually exclusive nor are they static; they may both exist for some people at different points in their illness experience; 'with each episode, another physical loss. With each event, another possibility of knowing self' (Charmaz, 1991: 258). Charmaz notes that not all people are able to achieve transcendence; not everyone has the insight, opportunity or motivation to do so. Other people are only able to do so in hindsight, having space and time to understand the personal meaning of their illness and re-shape their sense of self in response. There is ample evidence in our own data of the ways in which people actively and more implicitly sought to 'transcend' their illness and its effects, but there were also those people for whom transcendence was not an option and would not necessarily, had the option been available, be a choice they would make. Although Charmaz (1991) presents the notion of transcendence as a desirable, although perhaps unobtainable, state of being, it is necessary to temper this perspective, as we noted in the previous chapter, with one that recognises that, for some people living with chronic illness, the notion of transcendence or 'coming to term with' one's illness can constitute a particular form of tyranny. It can be an expectation, perhaps held by others, that it is possible to override the impacts, losses and disruptions caused by illness and that, to not do so, is a further indicator of personal failing – something those living with autoimmune conditions are all too familiar with in the context of everyday life and one that it is painful to have underlined when illness becomes overwhelming.

> The hardest lesson to learn from RA is that life preserving forces ravage us, putting an end to endless possibility.
>
> (Felstiner, 2007: 49)

Nonetheless, for some people, the journey to transformation, or, to couch the notion in specifically autoimmune terms, to reconstitute the conditions of self-tolerance, was an important facet of their illness experience. Embracing and learning from illness and assuming a positive attitude while accepting the limitations illness presents were common threads throughout people's narratives. For some, this was a self-imposed approach, while, for others, other people impelled them maintain a positive outlook, often in the face of great adversity.

> **Amanda:** Lupus is part of my life, it can be difficult but it has taught me so many valuable lessons too. I like my lifestyle now; accept myself and would like to train as a counsellor.

> **Shula:** Positivity… positivity… positivity… that is what I live by now. It is what enables me to keep going day by day and stretch myself that little bit further on the path to regaining my life back as it used to be. It's been a very long difficult road… having and living through what I have with lupus has taught me to be thankful for every day and count all my blessings and always look at the good things in life and not the bad. When I am having a bad day, I always tell myself there are so many people much worse off than myself – and I am so thankful for my LIFE.
>
> I've been told to stay positive and I try to tell myself that, but during the worst days of the illness this can feel futile and it can feel like an uphill struggle. I'm still learning!

What this evidence of biographical rehabilitation helps illuminate is the various ways in which people engage in biographical work to dress the assault on the self that autoimmunity (literally, or at the very least, biologically) constitutes. This work, reflected in the narratives above, focuses on: first, a refusal to change in the face of illness; second, the ways in which it is possible to 'unbecome' – to become a 'non-person'; third, to change completely, to become something one no longer recognises as self; or, finally, to integrate the effects of illness into one's self concept and come to a place of restitution and relative acceptance. There will, of course, be many other ways people manage illness in this sense, but, an overriding issue for us, is that biographical work in an autoimmune context is of a different nature to that undertaken in other illness. The very notion of autoimmunity, therefore, serves as an explanatory tool in coming to shape a sense of themselves (particularly for Ola in the previous quote). To re-invoke her words…

Throughout my childhood I suffered extensive abuse at home and at school. My mum didn't want a girl and throughout her life she continued to tell me I should never have been born and that having me had ruined her life. So I was physically fit, but mentally destroyed inside, with very low self-esteem and constantly under verbal attack within my family. Hardly surprising then that my immune system eventually joined in the attack.

Ola is effectively saying, here, I have become allergic and resistant to myself; a statement that is, surely, particular to the autoimmune experience. Her biographical work has involved refiguring her social and existential self in the face of illness, but this work also demands and imposes an ongoing biological vigilance, a perceived need to survey and monitor illness and potential deterioration.

## Mapping the autoimmune body

Foucault's (1973) work on the construction of the medical gaze has been well rehearsed and explicated in the literature on the sociology of health and illness.[2] 'The clinical form of panopticism' (Pryce, 2000: 105) and contemporary practices of clinician, health-related surveillance are part and parcel of our understanding of the social construction of health and disease. So too is our recognition of the way in which the 'individual is recruited into the modern project of self-observation' (Vaz and Bruno, 2003: 274). Maintaining health, anticipating and monitoring illness involves a perpetual process of self-surveillance and self-discipline, which means individuals accepting restrictions on their behaviour in order to care for their health even, and principally, when they may experience well-being (Vaz and Bruno, 2003: 274). Lupton (1995, 1999) suggests that such surveillance generates categories of individuals who are 'at risk' of illness or 'patients before their time' (Jacob cited in Vaz and Bruno, 2003: 274). The notion of the 'risky self', indeed the object of surveillance, involves us all as potential purveyors of illness and disease. Pryce (2000: 104) argues that 'surveillance is relocated through the individual citizen's observation of their "self" for signs of contamination, disease or dysfunction within cultures increasingly constructed as morally, socially, environmentally and biologically dangerous or "risky"'. Drawing on the work of Lupton (1999), Pryce (2000) suggests that the recruitment of, and self-examination by, the 'active patient' is central to governmentality and the construction of a new healthy citizenship, and that it arguably underpins current policies of self-care and self-management. Pryce's (2000) work demonstrates the extent to which regimes such as breast or testicular self-examination and, more latterly, aspects of surveillance embedded in the use of tele-care, are being routinely incorporated into everyday techniques of self-surveillance. Self-monitoring is a disciplinary mechanism of biomedicine, enacted in part in a discretionary manner. We are thus engaged with monitoring our own bodies to identify early signs of unpleasant, potentially life-threatening conditions. We are then in the business of identifying imagined risk and accorded the responsibility of monitoring and avoiding potential threats (Pryce, 2000) and keeping those that prevail at bay.

The lived experience of body surveillance and body-watching is an ongoing reality of monitoring long-term conditions, where risk is perpetual and monitoring an unwelcome act of perpetual self-discipline and fear. The continual anticipation of a return to, or deepening of, illness by people who are living with cancer, for example, is a well-researched phenomenon. Paul Stoller (2004: 192–193) writes about his own remission thus:

> Remission can also be like a prison from which the cancer patient cannot escape. Remission has been difficult for me… If I have a twinge in my abdomen, I fear that lymphoma cells are again on the rampage. If an ingrown hair causes a bump to develop in my armpit, I think it may be a swollen lymph node – another sign of lymphoma. If the flu makes me sweat at night, I worry that this too is a sign that cancer has returned. When I get a CAT scan every six months I wonder if my time is up…

In similar ways, several respondents in our study spoke of feeling compelled to continually map, search and watch for bodily changes. They spoke of living, not in remission, but in anticipation of illness, of 'turbulences' and living in the spaces between everything that has happened and what may continue to happen (Vaz and Bruno, 2003). Self-surveillance and policing their bodies, for new and worsening symptoms, effectively becoming a 'diseased body', accompanied the daily experience of living with lupus. Some people were preoccupied with the shifting physiologies and minutiae of their bodily changes, not least in the context of the side-effects of medication (McElhone et al., 2010; Mendelson, 2006). In the context of autoimmune conditions that are progressive, where the deterioration of the body is inevitable, body-watching is a technique of monitoring change but also a daily reminder of the permanency of the disease.

> **Martha:** Sometimes there are no changes at all, or no visible ones anyway, my body plateaus and the route into my disease is the regular blood tests I have, which provide a regular account of where my disease is up to at that moment. But there are times when I see my joints changing, sometimes in minutes its seems and the terrifying thing is that the swelling might change a bit but it doesn't go away entirely, Sometimes, the changes are incremental, I look down at my feet and think, the gap between my big toe and the next one never used to be that big but now it is unmissable. A space that continues to widen over time. Footwear, completely incidental for years, has never seemed so important! So a sore joint is not just a sore joint, it becomes a permanent state of being, a reminder of what is going on inside, which seems unstoppable.

This quote, while clearly illustrating the notion of body-watching, also speaks of an uncertain future where the disease process takes on a life of its own, becoming implacable and unstoppable.

## Uncertain futures

The lack of certainty illness can impose on the life course was a central concern for many of our respondents – the ways in which the future is planned, hoped for, envisioned and enacted. In a life without illness or other significant ongoing adversity, the future is ordinarily a place of hope, possibility and expectation. For those living with autoimmune conditions, however, it is a place also characterised by profound uncertainty, its shape being drawn and governed by forces often very much outside the person's control. In the midst of a lupus flare or when other illness is at the forefront of experience, many people found thinking about the future daunting and distressing. Under these circumstances, some people found that simply living one day at a time was the only way to manage the uncertainty that the future offered.

> **Pamela:** ... and during that time I was going through quite a bad time as well and she [doctor] was saying you just take each day, do what you can on that day and just each day, don't think ahead or back, just take each day. So that's what I do.

> **Molly:** You take things day to day, you know, it's a bit like somebody to say oh we'll go some, somewhere in a couple of months' time and you think I can't work that far ahead, I go from week to week, you know, we don't plan anything that far ahead because if you do and something happens, you know, but yeah, we go from week to week basically.

While this quotation suggests the need to live day-to-day and week-to-week, not consciously planning for the future, it also speaks of regret and the dismay that an uncertain future manifests.

The nature of lupus means that it is not possible for anyone with the diagnosis to hope or plan for a future without illness. As such, the horizons of chronically ill people are more distant and also less well-defined than might be the case for those living without ongoing ill-health.

> **Sharon:** You cannot plan because you... don't know, when it strikes you, how long it's going to last.

> **Victoria:** ... what we're trying to say is we don't put all the plums of life into the future because you don't know, you don't know what your future's going to be, you can't predict it.

Some people found that employing a micro-planning approach to daily activities in order to forestall predicted difficulties was a preferred technique for managing the unmanageable.

> **Gina:** I think ahead all the time now and I think, you know... I'll do this because if the pain increases then, you know, I'll be comfortable in this chair, or if I get my bedroom just right that, you know, I haven't got far to go from that point

to that point, I organise the garden that I haven't got a lot of walking from one chair, one seating area to another seating area.

The part of the future horizon for this person would seem to be the next daily challenge, the move from room to room and the topography of her immediate environment. In a similar context, maintaining a routine was seen as a way of managing pain and uncertainty.

**Moira:** I have to have a daily routine otherwise I will get worse. It does get a bit monotonous but it is for the best. I've worked out when's best to have a shower, do some reading, get caught up with friends, have a rest and go for a walk, and I have to stick to this. I'm still trying to work out how to adapt when something in that routine goes off and I am desperately trying to work out how I can be spontaneous and do something completely unexpected. I do set myself a task every day and I aim to do it, even if it is only having a shower before going back to bed.

The future, for these people in particular, was something that was either so indistinct or, conversely, frighteningly clear, that it was best ignored or at least disregarded.

**Nicki:** ... it's not a nice thought [ongoing illness] either is it, you know, if you think that, that could loom in your future? It's not something you really want to spend lots of time dwelling on. Not, not me anyway, I don't, no...

I don't want to let it in, so I suppose I am quite afraid of it really even though it sounds like it's probably just false bravado but I am, it does worry me and if I sit and think too long I think oh crikey, you know, all this horrible stuff that you hear about, no, that's not going to happen to me, no, cripes, just push that back there and leave it there although I know the truth of what it could be, no you're right, I do ignore it and push it away and not let it be part of me.

**Andrew:** Why worry about something until you actually know what you've got to worry about, just pointless... it's just a complete waste of energy and emotions, if someone says to you you've got x and perhaps then you start to get concerned before, there's no point getting concerned you might have it, because that's... just a waste of time, just stick it out the way and wait until the time comes.

Strategies aimed at challenging the bleakness of the future were commonly framed around the notion of positivity and maintaining a positive outlook, even, for some people, in the face of overwhelming difficulty.

**Dilys:** I do think anyone can develop a positive mental attitude with practice. I am not saying that I don't have my down days or moments when I feel sorry for myself, as I do, although now less frequent than before. I am currently doing some research into the way the mind works and the body's natural energy force. I do feel, however, that to tell yourself a positive action for the day to help you through it can really help with being more positive for the future. 'I can' and 'I will' are things I use all the time.

It is very easy to think your life is over and 'what is the point I will probably die soon anyway?'. By taking one day at a time and by looking in the mirror each morning and being thankful to have that day at all, really gives you the strength and encouragement to get through anything life has to throw at you. You master that and you can master anything.

I firmly believe (call me crazy if you like) that you become what you feel and think. If you think something bad will happen to you and you think it often enough and fear it, the chances are something bad will happen. If you think positive things then positive things will happen.

Making the most of the present, accepting what you have and being thankful were also common themes in this context.

> **Sharon:** I'd got some literature that basically said I was going to be dead in five years and I thought well if that's the case I've got to make the most of it, you know [laughs]. I'm just going to carry on, I'm going to do my teacher training and... I'm going to live, so that's what I did, got myself a job in Northumberland.

> **Sue:** ... we would do things rather than wait until I'm sort of 60, I mean I'm 55 just, so thought no I won't wait until I retire and I know I've got work until I'm 65 now, so technically. No, we're not going to wait... we're not silly, we're not in debt, so we're just, you know, do what we want to do sensibly when we want to do it, you know, because we don't know what's round the corner.

> **Victoria:** ... that is a good thing about having a chronic illness if you like, I've always, or we've always done what we wanted to do right then, I've always said do it now, you don't know what's going to happen.

For young people, in particular, living with the onset of an autoimmune condition can be particularly challenging and cruel when expectations and anticipations are uncertain and are forced into question. Future hopes and aspirations, in this context, are difficult to generate in the ways in which other young people may take for granted. It was, for the young people in our study, the manner in which the mundane became exceptional that was a particularly frustrating aspect of living with illness. There was also a sense that planning for the future and for the onset of symptoms was another aspect of living with illness that would not occur to the average young person.

At various points in her interview, Alice spoke at length about her vision of the future with lupus.

> **Alice:** I think a lot more about my future and stuff now, whereas I think most kind of 19-year-olds, they're just at uni kind of having a laugh and stuff but I do think a lot more about my future.
>
> Yeah, it is, it's hard because like I want to be going out and doing all things with my friends and stuff but... if there's a lot going on I have to think oh I'll go to that and I won't go to that because... I can't go out like, have late nights probably more than

like once or twice a week even because I just get so tired and if I get too tired then I just, I get really run down and I get poorly, so, yeah, I do have to pace myself.

This young woman was in her first year of university when we interviewed her. She had decided to remain at home for the duration of her first year at least, being uncertain of the impact of moving away, as many of her friends had done. This decision, again, was predicated on the unpredictability and management of her illness.

> ... whether or not that will actually affect me without me knowing, but, like my mum and dad said, I probably would have had to have moved anyway just because like hospital appointments and I'll get ill quite a lot and probably wouldn't really cope living on my own, right. This year, since September, like, like I say... with my sickness and stuff... I'd have been at home constantly anyway, so like it's hard because there's not really much point paying all that money if I'm going to be at home all the time anyway but then [it] might be the best thing I ever did, but I've decided not to this year because I am so settled here and enjoying it, I think it'd be a shame to maybe... risk it and then not be happy... but I think it has probably, like I do need more support so I don't think it'd work if I was miles away.

For Alice, and many others in our study, lupus became a key determinant in the trajectory of critical life decisions and, given that it is an evidently gendered condition, the experience of pregnancy and having children (and, for many women with lupus, miscarriage) was also a very visible theme in our data. This, again, is an ordinary life event that is imbued with additional complexity due to the nature of lupus and its associated effects.

> **Victoria:** ... had trouble conceiving, had a miscarriage.

> **Nicki:** I did read up about it and we thought well, you know, we'll try and if I'm going to have lots of miscarriages we'll probably either look, you know... alternatives really, maybe adoption or, or whatever but we'll see... what happens and I had two pregnancies and two babies, so I was lucky.

> **Rachael:** I think that's probably why I didn't want children, I think that was quite a conscious decision, you know, during that early period [in the illness] that I perhaps shouldn't have children... whether or not I'd be more prone to miscarriage, I just didn't... it turned out ultimately that I couldn't have children naturally anyway because I had severe endometriosis... and I had blocked fallopian tubes as a result of that and ovarian cysts, all sorts of things, but I had sort of decided even before all of that that maybe this wasn't for me, maybe parenthood wasn't going to be something that would happen for me.

Andrew, referring to friends who had lost a daughter to lupus, commented:

> ... their daughter, they've gone through hell, you know, she had three miscarriages, all caused by lupus, all three babies were fine, I'd forgotten they'd been

named and buried, and now they've got, their mother, their daughter, beside them, you know, they've got four graves in a row, that's not, that's not good stuff.

It is easy to lose sight of the fact that lupus, in addition to being incurable, can be life-limiting in the most literal sense. While there are some anticipated life events that are disrupted or absent because of lupus, there are others that are fundamentally accelerated. Living with lupus, like any autoimmune condition, is something of a lottery. There are no predetermined or predictable outcomes, the disease is the archetypal shape-shifter in the world of chronic illness, keeping one guessing at all times. The effects of this uncertainty are, in themselves, particularly challenging to live with and manage.

It is this uncertainty that, as we have variously noted, occupies the centre of the autoimmune experience and, as we have demonstrated in this chapter, the shifting sands of lupus are navigated on a variety of levels. This is the nature of lupus and the enduring flavour of the autoimmune experience. People map, navigate and understand this journey very differently, the multiple waypoints being determined variously by their pre-illness identity, their enduring and changing sense of self, the severity of their condition and the nature and extent of the support they are able to access – in this context, the variables that determine the nature and outcome of an individual journey are many and varied. What links each experience of autoimmunity, however, is an evident disjuncture between the pre- and extant-illness self that may be abrupt or more subtle. We would suggest, however, that the autoimmune paradox remains irreconcilable. This is despite the mechanisms that people might employ to engage in the biographical work necessary to live with an autoimmune condition and long-term illness more generally (practitioners employ immunosuppressants in an effort to reconstitute the self, for example, while patients engage in transformative quests for restitution). Ultimately, however, these efforts are inevitably overshadowed by the perpetual tussle between 'self and non-self'.

This work – and the struggles it represents – is undertaken in a variety of public, private and virtual spaces and it is to these different contexts that we turn in the following two chapters. First to the world of online illness, then, in Chapter 7, to the more intimate world of family relationships.

## Notes

1  Anderson and Mackay (2014).
2  See for example, Armstrong (1983, 1993, 1995); Nettleton (1995); Lupton (1994, 1999); Peterson and Bunton (1997).

## References

Anderson, W. and Mackay, I. R. (2014) *Intolerant Bodies: A Short History of Autoimmunity*. Baltimore: John Hopkins University Press.

Armstrong, D. (1983) *Political Anatomy of the Body: Medical Knowledge in Britain in the Twentieth Century*. Cambridge: Cambridge University Press.

Armstrong, D. (1993) 'From Clinical Gaze to Regime of Total Health'. In A. Beattie, M. Gott, L. Jones and M. Siddle (eds), *Health and Wellbeing: A Reader*. Basingstoke: Macmillan and Open University Press.

Armstrong, D. (1995) 'The Rise of Surveillance Medicine'. *Sociology of Health and Illness* 7(3): 393–404.

Charmaz, K. (1991) *Good Days, Bad Days*. New Brunswick: Rutgers University Press.

Felstiner, M. (2007) *Out of Joint: A Private and Public Story of Arthritis*. Lincoln: University of Nebraska Press.

Foucault, M. (1973) *The Birth of the Clinic: An Archaeology of Medical Perception*. London: Routledge.

Lupton, D. (1994) *Medicine as Culture: Illness, Disease and the Body in Western Societies*. London: Sage.

Lupton, D. (1995) *The Imperative of Health: Public Health and the Regulated Body*. London: Sage.

Lupton, D. (1999) *Risk*. London: Routledge.

Mendelson, C. (2006) 'Managing a Medically and Socially Complex Life: Women Living with Lupus'. *Qualitative Health Research* 16(7): 982–997.

McElhone, K., Abbott, J., Gray, J., Williams, A., and Teh, L.S. (2010) 'Patient Perspectives of Systemic Lupus Erythematosus in Relation to Health-related Quality of Life Concepts'. *Lupus* 19: 1640–1647.

Nettleton, S. (1995) 'Protecting a Vulnerable Margin: Towards an Analysis of How the Mouth Came to be Separated from the Body'. In A. Beattie, M. Gott, L. Jones and M. Siddle (eds), *Health and Wellbeing: A Reader*. Basingstoke: Macmillan and Open University Press.

Peterson, A. and Bunton, R. (eds) (1997) *Foucault: Health and Medicine*. London: Routledge.

Pryce, A. (2000) 'Frequent Observation: Sexualities, Self-surveillance, Confessions and the Construction of the Active Patient'. *Nursing Inquiry* 7: 103–111.

Stoller, P. (2004) *Stranger in the Village of the Sick: A Memoir of Cancer, Sorcery and Healing*. Boston: Beacon Press.

Vaz. P. and Bruno, F. (2003) 'Types of Self-surveillance: From Abnormality to Individual "at risk"'. *Surveillance and Society* 1(3): 272–291.

# 6    Digital illness

Autoimmune conditions affect approximately 10 per cent of the adult population (Department of Health, 2011). They are, as this book has shown, many and varied and some of them are particularly challenging to diagnose. The difficulties of diagnosis and the paucity of readily available information on rare autoimmune conditions in particular, means that contemporary technologies have necessarily become a major source of information, education and support. Indeed, some autoimmune conditions, such as lupus, are characterised by large, global, online patient communities. The ubiquity and centrality of the internet and digital health technologies thus critically construct, refract and orchestrate contemporary experiences of health and illness (Kivits, 2013).

In this context of a 'developing age of digital health' (Kivits 2013: 224; Lupton 2013, 2014), this chapter points to the ways in which many long-term conditions, and autoimmune conditions in particular, have become digitally mediated illnesses. The online environment, we suggest, facilitates the development of an 'autoimmune' digital identity, expressed in part, through a digital language – participants are 'lupies', 'spoonies', 'scleros/sclerodermians', 'fibros' and their practitioners, 'rheumies', all operating in an illness space referred to as the 'spooniverse'. It is the experience of digital technologies in the lives of some people living with autoimmune conditions and the multiple sources of support they turn to that are the primary focus of this chapter, which is written in two parts. The first outlines the development of the 'digital turn' in health and illness. The second explores how and why people use the internet and what the consequences of that use may be. Here we focus, in particular, on the construction of digital identities and 'netiquette', the ways in which illness is understood and expressed and how this shapes access and acceptance into the relevant online community.

## Tracing the dimensions of the digital turn in health

According to the Office of National Statistics (2013), 36 million adults (73 per cent) in Great Britain accessed the internet every day in 2013 – 20 million more than in 2006 and, of this number, 43 per cent used the internet to access health information.

> In 2007, approximately only one in five adults (18%) used the Internet to access health information using websites such as NHS direct. In 2013, 43% of all adults

had used the Internet to find health information online. Among those aged 25 to 34, the rate of use increased to nearly 6 in 10 (59%).

(Office of National Statistics, 2013: 5)

In the same year, just over half (53 per cent) of all adults used social networking sites. This use is not confined to younger age groups. 'One in every two adults (50%) aged 45 to 54 now report that they partake in social networking' (Office of National Statistics, 2013: 7). The figures follow a similar pattern in the USA. A health survey in September 2012 that explored how adults in the United States use the internet and digital technology for health and healthcare found that '81% of US adults use the internet [up to 86% in September 2013] and 59% say they have looked online for health information in the past year' (Pew Research Internet Project, 2013). Additionally, '35% of US adults say they have gone online specifically to try to figure out what medical condition they or someone else might have' and '72% of US adults living with chronic conditions have used the internet' for health-related reasons (diagnosis, monitoring, etc.) (Pew Research Internet Project, 2013), while Yahoo have reported that there are in excess of 2,000 online groups that focus on health-related issues (Bollier, 2010).

Digital technologies are clearly an integral part of daily life in the UK and elsewhere and are increasingly centrally implicated in the experience of health and illness. This shift, the 'turn' toward a digital experience of health and illness shapes the nature of medical practice and the experience of being a patient. Nettleton (2004: 661) suggests that, as a consequence, it is possible to identify a 'new medical cosmology'. Drawing on the work of Jewson (1976) and Armstrong (1995), she extends their typology of the social organisation of medicine, from bedside medicine (the first cosmology) to include 'e-scaped medicine'. This new cosmology outlines and frames contemporary medicine's engagement with the impact of digital technologies on medical knowledge and medical practice, scrutinises the nature of professional expertise and questions the trust which underpins it, thus demanding a re-examination of the relationship between patients and professionals (Nettleton, 2004). As Nettleton (2004: 676) argues, the 'escaping' and 'e-scaping' of medical knowledge shapes, 'social relations between practitioners and patients, medical education, medical practices, and indeed medical knowledge itself [which is] being transformed in ways which accord with the new scapes, opportunities and exchanges of information'. Illness-related information and knowledge has 'e-scaped' the traditional boundaries of the consulting room and the clinic, fast-flowing and leaking into easily accessible and increasingly influential spaces. The impact of the internet on the doctor/patient relationship in particular is most significant and has been a central research focus for health sociology and medicine, with both disciplines seeking to understand the ways in which power relationships are reformed and reconstructed within the new cosmology. Notwithstanding the limitations of the internet, some of which derive from inequalities of access on the basis of social class and geography, Hardey (1999: 401) has suggested that the internet heralded the possibility of transforming the doctor/patient relationship: quite simply, doctors no longer hold a monopoly over medical knowledge and the way in which it is accessed and utilised. Patients are, in effect, empowered by the internet (Kivits, 2013). The patient, in this context, becomes a co-producer of knowledge and an increasingly critical consumer of medical information and expertise (Hardey, 2001). Nettleton et al. (2005: 973) refer to this as a 'celebratory and empowering' approach, 'because of the supposed potential that the technology has for recalibrating power relations between patients and health professionals'. The internet, from this perspective, is part of a 'democratising impulse', a process of deprofessionalisation (or even cyberliberation) propelled by the development of patient expertise (Barker, 2008; Broom, 2005; Nettleton et al., 2005; Pitts, 2004). Gage and Panagakis (2012: 444) similarly identify the internet as providing 'patients with quick, unfettered access to a broad range of health-related information and support, and this access [has largely] contributed to the shift from physician-as-expert to patient-as-consumer healthcare encounters'. The expert patients that result are seen as self-advocates and equal participants and decision-makers in their management and care. Moreover, the internet can become a site of collective action and resistance. Rose (2007) and Nettleton et al. (2005) among others, cite resistance to vaccinations and HIV/AIDS activism as examples of this.

Nettleton et al. (2005) and Kivits (2013) outline the perspective of the medical profession as being in sharp contrast to this celebratory approach. The concerns expressed by the medical profession relate first to the quality and accuracy of information. Secondly, professionals have voiced doubts about lay people's (in)ability to make informed judgements about that information. The rise of technologies has also driven the increase in what might be termed unhelpful health-related behaviours, generating a range of new and unforeseen potentially problematic issues, not least the rise of what has been termed 'cyberchondria', the clinically unfounded anxiety generated by online symptom checking – stories of a person with indigestion surmising that they have an aortic aneurism are not at all uncommon.

Eysenbach and Kohler (cited in Kivits 2013: 217) demonstrated in their work that 'internet users do not have the competencies required to assess the accuracy of information and [tend] to scan information without evaluating the reliability of websites and their publishers'. The perception of the internet, then, as a tool for health information was a largely negative one: a view which, Kivits (2013) argues, to some extent still pertains. Nettleton et al. (2005: 874) suggest, however, that this polarisation of perspectives is unhelpful. Rather, they identify an 'emerging concordance between the lay use of the internet for health and illness and dominant (generally) biomedical conceptions of what constitutes "good quality" health information'. They argue that information sought online is used to supplement (and complement) that provided by health practitioners and, moreover, that people do not want to take full responsibility for diagnosis, managing and suggesting a prognosis for their illnesses. Rather, they still want to rely and draw on professional expertise, as they have historically done. Their study of people's use of online health information showed the use of what they refer to as 'rhetorical devices', which their respondents used to determine which information was trusted and which was not. Their research showed that 'real', respected organisations were primarily identified (in a virtual environment); UK websites and individuals were trusted more, as were non-commercial enterprises; sources considered professional were seen to be more trustworthy and personal opinion was not regarded as highly as professional knowledge. Finally, replication of information served to confirm its validity (Nettleton et al., 2005). This research points to the limitations of the 'empowerment' perspective. It confirms 'that the place of dominant medical practices and discourses remains [secure] in the culture of the information age' (Nettleton et al., 2005: 989) and asks us to consider the notion of 'concordance' in understanding the ways in which health information is accessed online. This position is reflected in Seale's (2005) broader analysis of internet usage where he shows that online information is organised in ways that mirror conventional, orthodox socio-economic power relations.

Broom's (2005) study of medical specialists' views on the impact of internet-informed patients provides a further perspective to that of 'concordance' or 'empowerment within limits' (Armstrong et al., 2011). His study showed that some specialists were positive towards the internet-informed patient in part because this tends to relocate a degree of responsibility to the patient. An active patient was seen as a 'safer' patient and, paradoxically, a more compliant one (Broom, 2005). Others he interviewed saw it differently: a number of specialists perceived the internet negatively – it was overwhelming and created confusion. Interestingly, this negative perspective was presented as one that 'protected the patient' rather than the specialist and their specialist knowledge. In some contexts, then, doctor/patient roles can be seen to be renegotiated, as the empowerment/deprofessionalisation thesis suggests. For others, however, the internet-informed patient was problematic and practitioners sought to reassert their authority, and engaged in 'disciplinary practices' (the practitioner actively asserting their professional dominance on consultation situations) to do so (Broom, 2005: 333). Broom concludes:

> instead of viewing the internet as contributing to the deprofessionalisation of medicine (Hardey, 1999:335), it should be seen as producing a complex process of adaptation on the part of specialists… at the very least these results suggest that the impact of the Internet-informed patient may be much more complex than previously argued, and second, that notions of the Internet as a challenge or threat may in fact misrepresent the significant variation in how specialists are experiencing and responding to the health information revolution.
>
> (Broom, 2005: 333)

Rose (2007: 142), locating this discussion in the context of 'biological citizenship' more generally, speaks of the ways in which biological citizens can be made 'from above' where science itself is represented as unproblematic, locating misunderstanding or divergence with the citizens themselves or 'vectors "from below" [that] pluralise biological and biomedical truth, introduce doubt and controversy, and relocate science in the fields of experience, politics and capitalism'. In this context, the internet thus becomes a vehicle for the disempowered and voiceless. This is a particularly interesting point in the context of diagnoses such as fibromyalgia, the online presence of which is demonstrably assertive and confident – perhaps precisely because of the absence of a biomedical diagnosis.

If the internet has altered the ways in which we make sense of the doctor/ patient relationship, it is also actively reshaping the reach, influence and place of 'the medical' in everyday life. Barker (2008: 22) draws our attention to the ways in which the internet medicalises a wide range of experiences thus extending the 'medical gaze', which is at once repressive and emancipatory. Drawing on Conrad (2005), she says, 'the internet can also fuel consumer demand for medical solutions to a range of human problems'. People access the internet in pursuit of information about common symptoms and everyday personal troubles. The web, Barker (2008: 22) argues, provides them 'with seemingly endless detail about innumerable medical conditions, diagnoses, and treatments – many of which were previously unknown to the individual – to discuss with their physicians'. On the one hand, Barker (like Hardey and others) suggests this extensive information empowers the public, transforming the patient into 'reflexive consumers' (Fox et al., 2005), yet it simultaneously runs the 'risk of medicalizing experiences that would otherwise remain outside of medicine's purview' (Barker, 2008: 22). The digital patient thus only exists in tandem with the digital practitioner, these two digital identities being shaped in sometimes uncomfortable, yet inextricably bound, virtual and real-life spaces. It is when the one space shades into the other that problems (and possibilities) can arise when patient actually meets practitioner outside the virtual environment. As such, the expert patient paradoxically plays a role in shaping what may or may not be regarded as the business of medicine (and health). In a similar vein, Kivits (2013) draws our attention to the profile of people using the internet for health reasons. These users are carers, friends, family and those seeking information in an effort to remain well. Ferguson (2002: 555), for example, demonstrated that 'a net savvy person in the immediate kinship group [is the one that] does most of the searching… When a new illness is diagnosed in a "wired" family, patients or caretakers reach out electronically to inform friends and family.' The healthy and the sick are both users of the internet, which is central to the culture of health consumption, in which we are responsible for the maintenance of our own personal health. 'In short, the Internet is viewed as part of a new way of "doing health"' (Kivits, 2013: 220). The significance and reach of the internet, whether liberating, medicalising, authoritative, supportive or otherwise, for those experiencing ill-health or not, is without question – as we have previously suggested, health and illness (and particularly the rare autoimmune conditions we focus on in this book) are now very much digitally mediated. The potential advantages of embracing digitally mediated healthcare are clear – better health outcomes, better compliance with treatment regimes and better-informed patients, but these outcomes can only be effectively realised if both patient and practitioner are able to engage in the resultant changes effected in their 'roles' in the clinical encounter. For practitioners in particular, this engenders the necessity to relinquish a degree of power and autonomy that has traditionally characterised at least one side of the clinical relationship. In the context of autoimmune conditions, as we have previously suggested, this entails also embracing uncertainty and making evident the imprecise nature of the medical knowledge that underpins many autoimmune conditions.

Lupton (2013) analyses the ways in which the digitised patient, through the use of mobile technology (mHealth/mobile health), engages in self-tracking, 'self-quantifying' and policing the body. Body functions and indicators such as

> blood glucose, body temperature, breathing rate, blood chemistry readings, body weight, blood pressure, heart rate, sleep patterns, cardiac output readings, and even brain activity, can all be monitored using portable, wearable and internal sensors, woven into clothing or laminated onto ultrathin skin surfaces and placed anywhere on the body.
>
> (Lupton, 2013: 394)

Self-tracking and the continual collection of data that promotes personal responsibility for health is central to the discourses of health education and health promotion. As Lupton (2013: 397) says, 'self-tracking represents the apotheosis of self-reflexivity in its intense focus on the self and using data about the self to make choices about future behaviours… self-tracking offers users of such technologies a strategy by which they feel they can gather data on their health indicators as a means of avoiding illness and disease'. While this discourse is similar to those of 'empowerment and (patient) expertise', and the potential reconfiguring of self and the body on one's own terms through technology (specify, digital, mobile, etc.), Lupton (2013: 401) points to the potential tyranny of body monitoring and body watching. Self-tracking, she says, 'may also come to be experienced as a burden rather than a vital source of self-knowledge and empowerment'. The digital patient experience is also one that is increasingly monetised. Using the notion of the 'digital patient experience economy', Lupton (2014) points to the ways in which 'patients' opinions and illness narratives may be expressed in more diverse and accessible forums than ever before, but simultaneously they have become exploited in novel ways in the era of digital health. The accumulation of 'big data' in the name of research, improved medical treatment and individual health may render participants vulnerable to exploitation (Lupton, 2014) in the context of privacy, the non-consensual use of data and the variety of ways in which mining big data may, ironically, impact negatively on a person (Bollier, 2010; Groves et al., 2013; Wigan and Clarke, 2013).

The impact of the internet on the doctor/patient relationship and the questions this gives rise to around trust and where it lies, the issue of expertise, who has it and how it can become destabilised, in whose interests the self-management of health lies and with what economic and cultural consequences, are all questions that shape our understanding, and impact, of the digital turn in medicine and healthcare. The internet appears to have become very much a third party in the patient/practitioner relationship, such that the dyad that has traditionally dominated much of our understanding of the medical encounter is now, of necessity, an often computerised and digitally conducted triad. It has arguably become an inescapable and integral dimension of the contemporary experience of health and illness and we now turn our attention to the specific ways in which people, particularly those with rare autoimmune conditions, experience and use the internet for health-related support and information.

**'I'd like to say thank you to you all for your kind comments, I'd do a bashful emoticon thingy if I knew how!' Experiences of being an online citizen**

Referring again to Sontag's (2001) invocation of the kingdom of the sick, Edwards (2013) reminds us of the relevance of her insights in the context of ever-increasing sickness and chronicity. As we have demonstrated in this book, Edwards (2013: 5) similarly says: 'The statisticians and experts tell us that more and more of us do – or will – belong to that "other place".' The internet provides a critical and easily available context in which to explore, embrace and/or resist citizenship (in the kingdom of the sick). It provides an avenue through which 'biosocial communities' (Rose, 2007) come together – to seek recognition, support, validation, knowledge and/or engage in 'biomedical self-shaping' (Rose, 2007: 142), in ways that are simultaneously disabling and empowering.

## The internet as a source of information and support

As we have noted above, the internet has been identified by practitioners and patients alike as a vital medium for health education and health promotion and another important tool in the pursuit and promotion of self-care/management – potentially a 'bottom-up form of welfare' providing effective healthcare information and support (Burrows et al., 2000). For example, Lindsay et al. (2008) in a study of the use of ICT in the management of heart disease demonstrated that access to digital media may have increased participants' knowledge, facilitating the self-management of their disease. 'Participants found the Internet useful for increasing their knowledge of healthy eating, especially the fat contents of foods and trying out new recipes they found online' (Lindsay et al., 2008: 326). The importance of the internet in also facilitating networks of support and information (largely experiential) is also very clear. Ziebland et al. (2004), in a study of how cancer patients experienced the internet, show how they used it for both information and support. They went online, for example, before visiting their doctor to try and make sense of their symptoms; in the process of diagnosis and treatment, their respondents used it to corroborate doctors' information regarding treatment, to supplement information, to make sense of medical terminology, to understand what to expect from treatment and recovery, to demonstrate competence, seek support and raise awareness about their conditions. Ziebland et al. (2004: 5) demonstrate that patients 'displayed considerable caution and competence and described techniques (such as comparing different information sources) to ensure that they were not misled', a palliative, perhaps, to the anxieties practitioners have articulated regarding patients' abilities to disaggregate and distil 'good' and reliable healthcare information from that which, at best, may be less useful and, at worst, misleading and potentially dangerous. Coulson (2013) looked at how online patient support communities affected the experience of people with inflammatory bowel disease. Like Ziebland et al. (2004), Coulson's study also demonstrated the role of the internet in both providing information and emotional support. Coulson (2013: 2) identifies some of the benefits of internet support communities: its easy accessibility; time to compose responses; no difficulties with travelling; no barriers that might be imposed by socio-demographic variables; the fact that the visible effects of disease can remain hidden and its anonymity and scope – there is no limit to the numbers of people who can join. He also identifies some problems, which include assessing the quality of information, too much negativity and the absence of face-to-face interaction. Gage and Panagakis (2012), in a study of parents of paediatric cancer patients' use of the internet, identify a number of reasons why their participants did *not* use the internet. These include fear, uncertainty, overload and logistical barriers. However, clarification of treatment options and social support and networking were identified as useful.

The range of experiences of and responses to the internet as a source of information and support were mirrored by the respondents in our own study of lupus, some of whom reported being frightened by some of the information they encountered online.

> **Sophie:** I'd got some literature that basically said I was going to be dead in five years and I thought well, if that's the case, I've got to make the most of it, you know.

> **Rachael:** At first I think I thought my life expectancy was really reduced. I thought oh jeez and then a colleague at work said I've just read an article about lupus and it was terrible, you know, and I think the lack of information, nobody in my family had heard of this before and also because of how thin I had become and how devastating it had been initially, I thought oh God, maybe I'm not going to make it past, I don't know 40 or something. Initially it was quite depressing, yeah it was quite upsetting initially and you know, starting to think, am I going to get through this?

Lupus has a very particular online presence. It is ubiquitous, in that the popular perception of the condition has been generated and framed, not least, by television drama (see, for example, *House*), which has popularised, yet also satirised, the condition. It is something of an ironic point – that this rare condition is perceived to be so ubiquitous. Everyone thus has something to say about lupus, but with little real knowledge about what it is to live with the condition. Getting a diagnosis of lupus was a particularly alarming experience for many of our respondents who often turned immediately to the internet. Our respondents' experience did not indicate a desire to be part of an 'illness community' – rather, this citizenship was, for many, an unwelcome dimension and reflection of their condition

> **Harriet:** We came back to the internet [after seeing the doctor] and looked it up, which I think is the wrong thing to do. You think, my God, I am going to die, and a lot of it said like a five-year lifespan.

Alan, Harriet's husband, said:

> After researching, looking to see what lupus was all about, and the first thing you see is, oh lupus is that [disease which] your immune system is attacking this, this

and this and everything is breaking down and you know, you might not be here next week, that was horrifying, really rotten… and you couldn't understand and the more I read, the more Harriet read, the more concerned we got.

Bob, Sue's husband, said:

> The word lupus was mentioned and they kept her in hospital. So, course, I came straight home, straight on the laptop, lupus, I read all about it. Only the worst case scenarios seemed to be there. Of course, you read that and your wife has just been diagnosed with it, it puts the fear of you know what up you.

While Kerry, one of our younger participants stated:

> When my mum looked on the internet she was like God, you've got a death sentence, you've got this, you've got that, you're going to get this, you're going to get that. And the information she got off the internet at the time was so… because it wasn't explained fully… she called it a death sentence.

Lucy said that when she was first diagnosed she avoided looking at the internet directly, but her daughter looked for her and, in doing so, actively filtered out some of the unwelcome negative information.

> **Lucy:** The worse thing is the… American websites. They are quite scary. You know, I don't look and when I was first diagnosed I wouldn't look, I'd get [upset]. So my daughter said she would sign up for one of the groups that send out emails and information and just tell me the bits that were positive.

The internet was, for some respondents, a place that offered the possibility of information yet also a place to fear and to be avoided. This was particularly the case soon after diagnosis where people sometimes received very little information about a disease that they had simply never heard of.

On occasion, people were actively warned away from using the internet as a source of information by their doctors who, ironically, were less than forthcoming in terms of information themselves.

> **Lucy:** My consultant said to me, 'do not go on the internet'; some of the things you will read are horrendous.

One respondent also reported having information that they gathered from the internet dismissed by their consultant. It was assumed, they felt, that they did not possess appropriate research skills to discern relevant information from misinformation. Once having demonstrated appropriate competence and, indeed, professional research skills, it was reported that the consultant engaged more willingly in the conversation – further evidence of the medical profession's anxieties about the leakage of medical information into a difficult to control sphere that patient have easy access to. These anxieties reflect a perceived need to protect the patient from misinformation, but also relate to the issue of who has access to information and, by definition, who then has the right (and the right skills) to appropriately interpret and apply it.

A number of our respondents sought information online precisely because they felt it was otherwise inaccessible or unavailable. Lydia and Alice used the internet as a means of assuaging what they perceived to be the inadequacies of the consultation, seeking information and reassurance in a virtual space when none was forthcoming in reality.

> **Lydia:** I think the consultant I see thinks I exaggerate (or that is how he makes me feel!). Last time I went I told him in the morning it feels like I am having a heart attack, can't breathe properly, pains up and down my left arm – his answer was 'well that is part of it'. He didn't explain why it is happening, what's causing it, or if I should be concerned, so, once again, I referred to the internet for help – which I shouldn't have to do.

> **Alice:** When something happens I'm straight on Google... And my mum says don't get so obsessed, like stop getting obsessed with it, but like it's just strange because I will like occasionally get really strange things like sometimes I'll get a pain round my chest and I'll feel like it's really bruised and apparently that's to do with it but no one's ever told us that, we just figured it out for ourselves, but like if you go to doctors, yes, just deal with that, they kind of just fob you off.

The place of the internet in providing an avenue to give and receive support is well-documented (Ayers and Kronenfeld, 2007; Burrows et al., 2000; Hardey, 2002) – online support has proved to be vital in the context of many chronic conditions but perhaps this is even more critical when people face lesser-known conditions. Our data points to the ways in which people with rare autoimmune conditions, those with contested and stigmatised conditions in particular, seek access and support and sometimes entry into the communities that are built around their illness. Berger et al. (2005: 1825) for example, demonstrate that 'people with stigmatised illnesses are more likely to turn to the internet for health-related information (for psychiatric and non-psychiatric stigmatised illnesses) than those without stigmatised illnesses'. Gage (2013) similarly speaks of the concept of 'experientially similar others'. She shows the significance of social networks to parents of paediatric cancer patients, for example – it was network ties that people formed with each other (in this context, in waiting rooms, on wards and in hospital hall ways) that were most significant, and supportive. Drawing on the work of Thoits, Gage (2013: 50) argues, 'individuals who have experienced a similar life stress can offer specialised emotional sustenance and active coping assistance'. The online environment offers similar possibilities for networks of support, particularly where those networks are formed around rare and/or stigmatised conditions.

Indeed, lupus (and other rare autoimmune conditions) is characterized by large online global communities: communities that, in many ways, provide a home, offering membership/citizenship to a 'biosocial community' (Rose, 2007) – a home that becomes most important in the absence of wider social recognition and understanding, characteristic of little-known and contested conditions as well as those that might be considered stigmatised (Sillence et al., 2007). In this context, online communities provide a critical link to others facing similar experiences. In her study of electronic support groups (ESGs) and fibromyalgia, Barker (2008: 23) demonstrates that there is a 'proliferation of ESGs run for and by people experiencing medically unexplained symptoms'. She continues, 'participants suggest that ESGs provide valuable information and social support that significantly alleviate distressing symptoms and minimise the self-discrediting impact of living with a contested illness' (Barker: 2008: 23). Her analysis of an online site (lay created and maintained) Fibro Spot demonstrates the ways in which exchanges authenticated the existence and experience of fibromyalgia. She describes a sense of 'illness solidarity' among participants in the face of 'medical disparagement' – people on Fibro Spot sought out names of doctors more open to the possibility of fibromyalgia, in the pursuit of a 'biomedical diagnosis' – what Barker (2008: 31) refers to as a search for 'physician compliance'. In sharp contrast to the notion of patient compliance, participants sought out doctors who would recognise the primacy of embodied experience, and concur with their definition of the situation. While this is clearly a reflection of patient power in an online community it, ironically, is one that continues to accord primacy to biomedical perspectives, thus medicalising a series of experiences also associated with socio-economic, and personal conditions (Barker, 2005). While the participants in the ESGs in Barker's study arguably reify illness, the participants nonetheless, 'commiserate, collaborate and support one another' (Barker, 2008: 32). In doing so, they adopt a digital illness identity: one that validates their experience, confirms their symptoms and affirms their (sought) place in 'the kingdom of the sick'. Internet communities thus constitute biosocial entities that aid in the development of techniques for managing everyday life with chronic illnesses.

Approval and award of online 'biological citizenship' is however complex and contested. Online 'netiquette', personalities, behaviours and the ways in which illness is understood and expressed, shapes access and acceptance into online communities. The internet has come to constitute another forum in which the notions of 'bad', 'good' and 'expert' patient are particularly pertinent. In this context, Bar-Lev (2010: 147) suggests that the internet also acts as a 'moral space'. Rier (2007) provides an interesting example of this in a study that explored HIV+ status disclosure in internet social support groups. This study demonstrated the ways in which internet support groups can act as 'moral agents'. The ethics of disclosure in sexual relationships demonstrated this very clearly when responses to HIV+ people who posted comments that they had had unprotected sex elicited an angry response. For example, one woman posted a comment:

> My boyfriend has just asked me to marry him I love him very much and want 2 say yes but he doesn't know I'm positive and I can't bring myself 2 tell him 4 fear of losing him, any suggestions?
>
> (Rier, 2007: 1049)

Rier (2007: 1049–1050) presents a number of responses to this post, one of which he describes as a 'bitter attack', or as 'flaming' (writing in very sharp tones on the internet):

Ok so you had unprotected sex with the man you 'love' knowing that you could have infected him... and now you are looking for love and support from us and from him? If you can tell me you really believe you DESERVE love right now... I'll send you... heart shaped chocolates for every day of ur self absorbed life... Jesus lady, grow up, invest in some morals...

(Rier, 2007: 1049)

Rier (2007: 1053) argues that the online support groups do provide a forum for debating moral and ethical questions, but they are also forums that are self-monitored and policed – 'posters to AIDS lists police online discourse to mark and attack positions deemed immoral and dangerous'. He states that this resulted in some people shifting their position, for example, on HIV-status disclosure. Rier (2007: 1055) argues that the online forums which he explored 'functioned as clearinghouses for and transmitters of existing discourses' – there are 'appropriate' and 'inappropriate' ways of being an online citizen, it seems. As he concludes, 'clearly there's more to support groups than support'.

Further examples of what happens when a person contravenes the self-styled conventions and rules of an illness community are easy to find online. For contested illnesses in particular, people who do not demonstrate what might be termed the 'party line' of an illness community or who actively undermine its wider project are unceremoniously 'flamed' and singled out for particular negative attention. In a study of an online self-help group for Norwegian breast cancer patients, Sandaunet (2008) explores the reasons why people withdrew from the support group. In the same way that fear was the reason why people chose not to look at the internet for information, or to look only at very specific, largely medically sanctioned sites (see above), avoiding painful details about their illness was another reason cited. For example, one woman said she dropped out because she could not 'bear all the terrible stories':

I was recently diagnosed with this myself. To hear about all the problems and all the recurrences got too much. I had to quit and find information other places.

(Sandaunet, 2008: 135)

The women in this study sought other women online who they could speak to about survival. Other themes identified by the women were, 'not being ill enough' – women experienced the forums as places for others who were 'worse off than themselves' (Sandaunet, 2008: 136). This was identified as a reason for non-participation in support groups (virtual and otherwise) by some of the people who participated in our lupus study.

**Rachael:** I was contacted by a local lupus group and I was chatting to them about my lupus. [They said] you're working? Oh my goodness, it was like miraculous to them and I just thought I am not going to make contact with you on a personal level [to discuss my situation] because that would be depressing. My situation is not what they are targeting; they're targeting people whose experience of lupus is far worse off. I don't want to be involved in these networking groups, it's not for me. I don't want to talk about it every day, and I feel a bit fraudulent to do that as well, as I say, my condition is probably at the better end of the spectrum. From what I have seen of lupus on the internet, people are willing to talk about it and share, I'm just not going to be one of them.

The women in Sandaunet's (2008) study also said they felt pressure to report successful stories, and feared that they did not want to be seen as complaining, moreover the phases of their illness (remission and recovery) mitigated against participation. Veen et al. (2010) explore the ways in which patients with celiac disease used an internet support forum to manage the stringent dietary regimes required in controlling celiac disease. They demonstrate that dietary management is a collective rather than individual issue (Veen et al., 2010: 25). The support forum in this context acted as a bio-collectivity to encourage, people 'not to quit the diet'. Dietary compliance is then both a collective phenomenon as the authors suggest but it is also an example of 'moral agency'. One of their respondents posted the following comment:

> I am so fed up with this diet. I hate the fact that I have to think before I eat. Think before I eat. There is no freedom in that and it is making me angry, which is increasing my depression. Has anyone decided to bag it in and just go back to a gluten filled diet? What happened? I have been strictly gluten free since being diagnosed but I am ready to quit.
>
> (Veen et al., 2010: 29).

One person responded thus:

> I do get very frustrated and depressed at times. I feel like the disease has taken away my freedom to eat where I want, when I want, and not to read a label EVERY time I buy something. Having said that I have never cheated (I have been accidentally glutened). Not because I am perfect or live in a bubble, more because I found a will to stay gluten-free. For me it was my kids. If they someday get this disease I want them to see me as a positive example.

While this participant clearly empathises with the aggravation and anger evident in the initial post and shares her own sense of frustration at the dietary limitations imposed by celiac disease, there is also an attempt at providing a moral and/or altruistic rationale (her family) for maintaining her dietary compliance. The bio-collectivity of online support groups thus function as repositories and providers of support and advice (a welcome into a largely unwelcome world of illness), yet they are also spaces where 'moral work' is clearly evident – both on the part of lay participants and more formal moderators.

In a study of peer-to-peer discussions in a virtual diabetes clinic, Armstrong et al. (2011: 359) similarly found that individual community members 'negotiate and enforce the boundaries surrounding what could and could not be expressed'. Some members presented themselves as knowledgeable and authoritative, sanctioning, legitimising or challenging the validity of views expressed.

Julie spoke of some of the hostility she encountered in online lupus forums as her illness experience, particularly her diagnosis, differed markedly from the more usual diagnostic journey. Describing her depression she said,

> I felt utterly devastated about having lupus mainly due to reading some horrific (out of date) facts about how I would probably be dead within a few years. I then went through the 'why me, what have I done to deserve this' phase. Followed by separating from my partner (won't go into all the details but lupus did play a small part as he didn't take it seriously because I looked fine on the outside). Then followed a depression phase so I tried to talk to the others in the same situation on forums but I felt I had upset them by getting my diagnosis so quickly. This depressed me even more. I felt bad enough already without hearing about more ills and woes... online it seemed that long-term forum members would sympathise with new members who were struggling with getting a diagnosis [the more usual diagnostic journey], offering them tips and suggestions but I got the impression that I was being ignored, perhaps they felt like I didn't need help.

In a similar vein, Moira said:

> When I was diagnosed with fibro I tried the online boards but found them too depressing and it made me sort of guilty. I was responding really well to the amitriptyline and no one else was. I was able to have a bit of a life and they didn't. I very quickly gave up the online thing until just before my SLE diagnosis when I found Sara Gorman's blog (despitelupus.blogspot.co.uk). It was the first positive thing I read about lupus and here she was discussing similar emotions to what I was having. Fantastic.

While some people have clearly found the online environment hostile and less than helpful, the quality of the online experience being shaped by whether or not a person assumes the correct 'patient characteristics' – i.e., demonstrating the required and expected trajectory and profile of certain conditions, others have had a much more satisfying and reassuring experience (Armstrong et al., 2011). These varieties of experience, we would argue, are very much dependent on the internal politics of an online resource and the willingness of participants to adopt and fulfil required roles and responsibilities. The world of online illness is a space where communities generate their own particular hierarchies, where certain members, by virtue of their own illness status, are posited, and assume, the status of expert by experience. An apposite example of this is evident on the 'Inspire' scleroderma forum. Here, in addition to access to support from other people living with a rare autoimmune condition, there is a wealth of disease specific information that is generated from both experience and research. Even the most cursory reading of some of the forum's posts would persuade the reader that the medical profession, on the whole, is not familiar with the complexities of this rare autoimmune disease. On this particular forum, in addition to readily available complex clinical information garnered from a range of sources, there exist a number of highly influential and knowledgeable people: individuals who offer (with the necessary riders) clinical information and whom other members readily consult and defer to. We present this forum thread in some detail, as it illuminates a number of the key points we have referred to in this chapter.

A person enters the forum experiencing alarming symptoms and an equally distressing diagnostic encounter. Within a short time, support and an alternative reading of her symptoms and the diagnosis are forthcoming. The second poster is at pains to point out the value and limitations of the internet as a health information resource while Choclit (the third person to respond and a mainstay of this forum, being generally recognised as an expert by experience) has written a range of information materials for people diagnosed (and awaiting diagnosis) with scleroderma, which is very detailed, thoroughly researched and is often quoted as a seminal resource by many people using the forum (and beyond). He speaks with an authority readily underpinned by other contributors who are also keen to embrace a new member of the scleroderma 'family'. A sense of community and support is quickly generated and serves to allay the first poster's evident anxiety. Information is provided that is safe and reliable and support is forthcoming from others who are experiencing some of the same issues (perhaps the most telling sentence is the one in which the original poster 'TwoCatsWashing' is invited to join the scleroderma family, a select, if reluctant, grouping of disparate, yet similarly challenged, people). What this thread also offers is an insight into the speed with which the virtual world can provide reassurance and information. Within an hour of posting, 'TwoCatsWashing' is clearly feeling relieved and less anxious about her diagnosis.

**TwoCatsWashing** May 2, 2014 at 1:11 am

Hello, I was recently referred to a rheumatologist for Reynaud's symptoms, and in reviewing my blood panel he said that I showed I have scleroderma. I would return in 4 months and we would forego vasodialators at this time and reflux meds since I was not experiencing enough to want to go on a systemic at this point. I left the office knowing nothing more, and of course proceeded to get home and investigate scleroderma online. Frightening! Many things I thought were just old age starting to set in (I'm 48) were matching symptoms for systemic scleroderma, and the positive SCL-70 of over 8 and positive ANA was seeming ominous. Mortality in the 40% range at 10 years? What is this? I wrote my physician an email to please give me some more specifics…his reply: 'The Scl-70 is high and is most associated with diffuse systemic sclerosis. However, the presence of antibody is not an absolute determination of diffuse systemic sclerosis'. Ok… so now what? My family is begging for a second opinion. Meanwhile, my tight jaw, lump in my throat, sunburn feeling on my shins, out of breath periodically and general fatigue is alarming… I'm a licensed Veterinary nurse and understand medicine well, and from what I'm feeling/reading, the prognosis is not good. Doctors are loathe to give absolutes, but what I'd like is some honest feedback – what do I have in store? I want reality, not flimsy hope…will I see 15 yrs from now? Scared and alone…

**lynncrb1**
Reply 5218277

May 2, 2014 at 1:29 am

TwoCats, I just posted earlier on someone else's entry that a positive blood test does not mean you have any given autoimmune disease; if you made everyone take those tests many people would turn out positive and never get the disease. These diseases are incredibly difficult to diagnose and that's why it often takes years – you have to see how many other symptoms you get before you can say you have something. And of course once you're afraid you have something you start to think every new ache and pain is related to this disease you fear.

I am not saying that you don't have or won't get diffuse scleroderma, but even if you do, everyone has a different path they take and the problem with looking these diseases up online is that we often just read about worse-case scenarios. There are many people who have scleroderma who lead normal and productive lives with few symptoms – you just don't know! Like I said earlier, the Internet can give you great comfort but it can be a source of unnecessary worry.

I hope you feel better.

**Choclit**
Reply 5218741
May 2, 2014 at 8:43 am

You may find the draft version of my forthcoming 'Guide for New and Future Patients (and Their Families)' helpful. Note that it is currently under medical review so the specific recommendations on testing may change before it is released. Here is a link to that document:

http://www.sclerodermafaq.info/Guide_for_New_Patients.pdf

It is a companion document to my larger and more comprehensive document: 'Scleroderma FAQ'. The draft version of that document is located at

www.sclerodermafaq.info/Draft_6.pdf

Please follow up with any questions. There are a lot of helpful people on these forums. Finding a scleroderma specialist, as Rinnah suggested, is a good idea if that is a possibility for you.

**TwoCatsWashing**
Reply 5219476
May 2, 2014 at 1:02 pm

Wow, all I can say is thank you everyone… I went to bed confused and disheartened, and woke to all your answers feeling like I have hope, direction, and new friends. Blessings everyone for the gift you've given me… not false hope, but a real hope. Thank you, thank you, thank you.

**exotec**
Reply 5222076
May 3, 2014 at 1:34 pm

Hi 2cats! I'm a retired Vet Tech – and having that background and reading the info online can indeed induce fear and depression! But keep reading. Don't let those reports define how *your* sclero is going to manifest. It's uniquely different for each of us.

choclit has written a most excellent FAQ on it – far more complete than you're likely to find in any other resource. I strongly recommend you read that!

This is a great site to compare symptoms and management techniques. It helped me stop thinking of it as a 'death sentence', which was about where I was in the initial stages. I've seen reports here of people who have been living with sclero for many long years, and still have lives worth living. I stopped thinking in terms of how much longer it will let me live. I've decided I'm going to live to the fullest extent I can manage, for as long as I hope to do. So far, a positive outlook and determination have been crucial parts of my 'management'.

This isn't to say you can ignore it – it's a serious condition and must be managed enthusiastically (?) with your healthcare team. You have to be your own advocate. You must be an integral part of your therapy. And you already know how important histories and progressions or changes are to diagnostics and ongoing therapy. Start a journal – keep that diary of daily symptoms, feelings, reactions to meds… take that with you to every appointment and make notes of the office visit in it so you can refer back.

Meanwhile, be part of our 'family', because no one can understand this rare condition like we do. No one else can be there to support the bad days, nor rejoice in small victories as we will. Check in with us often. We're right there with you, each in our own way.

We have outlined the ways in which the online environment can both support and hinder the illness journey and, in our own study of lupus, we were surprised by the way in which people readily embraced the opportunity to talk and articulate their experience of illness through the virtual medium. Our research blog unexpectedly functioned in some respects like an online support group. Over a period of three months a total of 40–45 different people contributed 148 posts in four different threads. Some respondents corresponded with each other as well as ourselves as researchers. Some of their posts reflect the both the value and the pressures that arise in support groups. For example, Isabel was describing her symptoms and felt it necessary to apologise for the tone of her post:

> **Isabel:** Following a 4 week stint in January 2009 (It was so bad I could not move a muscle and actually at times wished I was not around) Apologies for the morbid undertones but I have never felt so low. It took nearly 6 months to start to recover from that stint in hospital. It was an infection they said. I managed to get a place at college to study architecture, was getting fit by swimming and was feeling quite positive despite losing my job and having to use crutches all the time. Then in November 2009, I had a heart attack while swimming. I'll sign off now before I get too morbid and frighten everyone off the blog. I'll be more positive next time.

A correspondence developed between two participants. One was responding to someone who had been struggling to get a diagnosis. They said:

**Chau:** I hope you get your diagnosis soon. If I could offer you any advice to aid this it would be to keep a diary, list all your symptoms, aches and pains daily and always take it with you to doctors appointments. Good luck for when you decide to return to work. I've been back two days now! If anything being at work for me is more peaceful and means less running around than being at home with the babies, only it's an awful lot less enjoyable and nowhere near as rewarding! Hope you get more sleep tonight.

Ruth wrote in response:

Thanks Chau, will keep a diary, that would really help, sometimes when I'm at the hospital I leave and wish I'd said more, so that should help, thanks. I'm going to get that book you mentioned too! Thanks for the advice, mixed emotions about returning to work, will be fine

The various excerpts and examples of online illness behaviours and identities we have presented here suggest that online 'biological citizenship' is fraught with challenges and possibilities (Rier, 2007) that reflect complex (digital) illness identities rooted in and reflective of medical, lay, expert-patient experience, knowledge and power. They, and the internet more generally, are an integral component of understanding and living with illness and, in the context of rare conditions such as lupus, can be a vital lifeline to information, recognition and support.

We have outlined the ways in which the internet is inseparable from and integral to experiences of health and illness for patients and practitioners alike. The evidence suggests that it is a potential tool of empowerment through which those thrust into illness, and others seeking to protect themselves from ill-health, can engage in making sense of their experiences in their own way and context. Yet, it is also clear that the internet, including securing regular access to it, is not distinct from, but rather embedded in, the everyday relations of power, knowledge and inequality that characterise the practice and social experience of medicine. In other words, the expert patient, involved in the self-management of their long-term condition/s will continue to defer to (and seek out) the voice and authority of biomedical medicine, albeit from the vantage point of information, support and the experience of others. While our illness can be experienced in, and reflected through, the virtual spaces of the internet, the fact remains that it is impossible to fully 'e-scape' the embodied nature of chronic illness. This, allied to the fact that we are obliged to access actual healthcare and support outside of the virtual world, means that it is not possible to escape our embodied selves or the bureaucratic, institutional ways in which it is provided and funded. Yet, the internet has made the experience of being a patient (and a doctor) much more complex. As such, the development of what might be termed the 'e-patient' and the ways in which the internet has democratised medical knowledge is radically redefining and reshaping the clinical relationship.

There is little doubt of the extraordinary possibilities that the internet promises for 'citizenship' – biological citizenship into the 'kingdom of the sick', which entitles the citizen to a voice (especially in the context of poorly understood, rare conditions), to knowledge and, critically, to support. Yet, this citizenship does not provide unfettered access or unrestrained opportunities to speak, for, like the experience of 'being a patient', in an everyday lived reality, this citizenship is characterised by hierarchical relations of power shaped by illness – its nature, form, duration, severity and future.

## References

Armstrong, D. (1995) 'The Rise of Surveillance Medicine'. *Sociology of Health and Illness* 17(3): 393–404.

Armstrong, N., Koteyko, N. and Powell, J. (2011) 'Oh Dear. Should I Really Be Saying That on Here? Issues of Identity and Authority in an Online Diabetes Community'. *Health* 164: 347–365.

Ayers, S. L and Kronenfeld, J. J. (2007) 'Chronic Illness and Health-seeking Information on the Internet'. *Health* 11(3): 327–347.

Barker, K. K. (2005) *The Fibromyalgia Story: Medical Authority & Women's Worlds of Pain*. Philadelphia: Temple University Press.

Barker, K. K. (2008) 'Electronic Support Groups, Patient-Consumers, and Medicalisation: The Case of Contested Illness'. *Journal of Health and Social Behaviour* 29: 20–36.

Bar-Lev, S. (2010) "Do You Feel Sorry for Him? Gift Relations in an HIV/AIDS On-line Support Forum'. *Health* 14(2): 147–161.

Berger, M., Wagner, T. H. and Baker, L. C. (2005) 'Internet Use and Stigmastised Illness'. *Social Science and Medicine* 61: 1821–1827.

Bollier, D. (2010) *The Promise and Peril of Big Data*. Washington, DC: The Aspen Institute.

Broom, A. (2005) 'Medical Specialists' Accounts of the Impact of the Internet on the Doctor/Patient Relationship'. *Health* 9(3): 319–338.

Burrows, R., Nettleton, S. and Pleace, N. (2000) 'Virtual Community Care? Social Policy and the Emergence of Computer Mediated Support'. *Information, Communication and Society* 3(1): 95–121.

Conrad, P. (2005) 'The Shifting Engines of Medicalization'. *Journal of Health and Social Behavior* 46: 3–14.

Coulson, N. (2013) 'How Do Online Patient Support Communities Affect the Experience of Inflammatory Bowel Disease? An Online Survey'. *Journal of the Royal Society of Medicine* 4: 1–8.

Department of Health (2011) *Improving NHS Services for Rare Autoimmune Diseases: A Review by the Independent Expert Clinical Group on Rare Autoimmune Diseases*, www.mhpc.com/wp-content/uploads/2012/09/Improving-NHS-services-for-rare-autoimmune-diseases.pdf (accessed 8 February 2013).

Edwards, L. (2013) *In the Kingdom of the Sick: A Social History of Chronic Illness in America*. New York: Walker Publishing.

Ferguson, T. (2002) 'From Patients to End Users: Quality of Online Patients Networks Needs More Attention than Quality of Online Health Information'. *British Medical Journal* 324(7337): 573–577.

Fox, N. J., Ward, J.K. and O'Rourke, A. J. (2005) 'The "Expert Patient": Empowerment or Medical Dominance? The Case of Weight Loss, Pharmaceutical Drugs and the Internet'. *Social Science and Medicine* 60: 1299–1309.

Gage, E. (2013) 'Social Networks of Experientially Similar Others: Formation, Activation, and Consequences of Network Ties on the Health Care Experience'. *Social Science and Medicine*. 95: 43–51.

Gage, E.A. and Panagakis, C. (2012) 'The Devil You Know: Parents Seeking Information Online for Paediatric Cancer'. *Sociology of Health and Illness* 34(3): 444–458.

Groves, P., Kayyali, B., Knott, D. and Van Kuiken, S. (2013) *The Big Data Revolution in Healthcare: Accelerating Value and Innovation*, www.mckinsey.com (accessed 9 April 2015).

Hardey, M. (1999) 'Doctor in the House: The Internet as a Source of Lay Health Knowledge and the Challenge to Expertise'. *Sociology of Health & Illness* 21(6): 820–835.

Hardey, M. (2001) '"E-Health": The Internet and the Transformation of Patients into Consumers and Producers of Health Knowledge'. *Information, Communications & Society* 4(3): 388–405.

Hardey, M. (2002) '"The Story of My Illness": Personal Accounts of Illness on the Internet'. *Health* 6(1): 31–46.

Jewson, N. D. (1976) 'The Disappearance of the Sick Man from Medical Cosmology 1770–1870'. *Sociology* 10(2): 225–244.

Kivits, J. (2013) 'E-Health and Renewed Sociological Approaches to Health and Illness'. In K. Orton-Johnson and N. Prior (eds), *Digital Sociology: Critical Perspectives*. Basingstoke: Palgrave Macmillan.

Lindsay, S., Bellaby, P., Smith, S. and Baker, R. (2008) 'Enabling Healthy Choices: Is ICT the Highway to Health Improvement?' *Health* 12(3): 313–331.

Lupton, D. (2013) 'Quantifying the Body: Monitoring and Measuring Health in the Age of mHealth Technologies'. *Critical Public Health* 23(4): 393–403.

Lupton, D. (2014) 'The Commodification of Patient Opinion: The Digital Patient Experience Economy in the Age of Big Data.' *Sociology of Health and Illness*.

Nettleton, S. (2004) 'The Emergence of E-scaped Medicine?' *Sociology* 38(4): 661–679.

Nettleton, S., Burrows, R. and O'Malley, L. (2005) 'The Mundane Realities of the Everyday Lay Use of the Internet for Health, and their Consequences for Media Convergence'. *Sociology of Health & Illness* 27(7): 972–992.

Office of National Statistics (2013) *Internet Access – Households and Individuals*, www.ons.gov.uk/ons/dcp171778_322713.pdf (accessed 24 January 2014).

Pew Research Internet Project (2013) *Health Online 2013*, www.pewinternet.org/2013/01/15/health-online-2013 (accessed 10 March 2014).

Pitts, V. (2004) 'Illness and Internet Empowerment: Writing and Reading Breast Cancer in Cyberspace'. *Health* 8(1): 33–59.

Rier, D. (2007) 'Internet Social Support Groups as Moral Agents: The Ethical Dynamics of HIV+ Status Disclosure'. *Sociology of Health & Illness* 29(7): 1043–1058.

Rose, N. (2007) *The Politics of Life Itself: Biomedicine, Power and Subjectivity in the Twenty-First Century*. Princeton: Princeton University Press.

Sandaunet, A. (2008) 'The Challenge of Fitting In: Non-participation and Withdrawal from an Online Self-help Group for Breast Cancer Patients'. *Sociology of Health & Illness* 30(1): 131–144.

Seale, C. (2005) 'New Directions for Critical Internet Health Studies: Representing Cancer Experiences on the Web'. *Sociology of Health and Illness* 27(4): 515–540.

Sillence, E., Briggs, P., Harris, P. R. and Fishwick, L. (2007) 'How Do Patients Evaluate and Make Use of Online Health Information?' *Social Science & Medicine* 64: 1853–1862.

Sontag, S. (2001) *Illness as Metaphor and AIDS and its Metaphors*. London: Picador.

Veen, M., te Molder, H. F., Gremman, B. and van Woerkum, C. (2010) 'Quitting is Not an Option: An Analysis of Online Diet Talk Between Celiac Disease Patients'. *Health* 14(1): 23–40.

Wigan, M. R. and Clarke, R. (2013) 'Big Data's Big Unintended Consequences'. *Computer* 46(6): 46–53.

Ziebland, S., Chapple, A., Dumelow, C., Evans, J., Prinjha, S. and Rozmovits, L. (2004) 'How the Internet Affects Patients' Experience of Cancer: A Qualitative Study'. *British Medical Journal* 328: 1–6.

# 7 Situating the family in the experience of chronic illness

In the previous chapters we have explored the changes that lupus and other auto-immune conditions impose on the practices of everyday life. Becoming and being ill, pre- and post-diagnosis, significantly shapes our identities, our expectations of ourselves and others, our life trajectories and, of course, our relationships – daily living is constituted in and through our relationships with others in the context of living with an autoimmune condition. We have looked at the complex relationships we share with medical practitioners, which are variously characterised by scepticism, ongoing tussles for legitimacy and authority, access to resources, warmth, understanding and a sense of critical support when it is forthcoming. Yet, it is our relationships with our children, parents, partners, lovers, siblings, friends and colleagues that mediate our experiences of illness on a day-to-day basis. It is to these fundamental relationships – the building blocks of our everyday lives, which shoulder the possibilities, consequences and responsibility for managing constant change and uncertainty – that we now turn. In so doing, this chapter explores the interaction between illness and relationships, and the changes, adaptations and reiterations it brings, imposes and offers.

Our primary focus in this chapter is the family, our starting point being to briefly examine the ways in which family has been considered in the health (policy and practice) literature on chronic/long-term conditions. Here we suggest two things; first, that 'family' appears to have been neglected or at very least has an 'assumed or presumed status', i.e., that everyone has 'a family' and that it will inevitably perform a support function. Further, that family is very often framed as a structured, reliable and inflexible entity that illness inevitably disrupts and unsettles. The family is a structure that absorbs and mediates the effects of illness. The family, from this perspective, we suggest, is a core (if largely unwritten) part of a health and social care system focused on the efficiency and cost-effectiveness required in the self-management/care of chronic, long-term conditions. We argue here that, while the focus on self-care is underpinned by patient expertise, partnership with practitioners, independence and empowerment – in other words a more obvious explicit, elucidative embracing of the social model of health – it ironically falls short of embracing the 'social'; family and its associated complexities remain largely absent in both the policy and practice of healthcare. Paradoxically, the voice of family members who are living with people with chronic conditions has never been more present, yet their experiences have also been abstracted from the notion of 'family', having been repackaged as 'carers'. Historically, the acknowledgment and formalisation of 'care', in part, derives from early feminist analyses of the gendered nature of family obligations, which also served to highlight the injustice of unpaid labour and the significant economic and social consequences of undertaking caring responsibilities (Twigg and Atkin, 1994). Arguably, the formalisation of 'care', for reasons of equality and economy, at opposite ends of the ideological scale, has served to abstract the family and its network of relationships from view, theoretically and in practice. In response to this individualised and medicalised understanding of the family, we suggest that family sociology, and its invitation to understand the family as a set of processes and practices, including its more recent focus on 'doing' (Morgan, 1996) and 'displaying' family (Finch, 2007) may further our understanding of how families experience and 'do' chronic long-term conditions. Our focus here is a very specific one. It is to suggest that 'family' relationships have been inadvertently marginalised either through the application of the biomedical model or, ironically, through the invocation of the concept of 'carer'. This, we suggest, is particularly apposite with those long-term conditions, such as lupus, rheumatoid arthritis and multiple sclerosis, which are characterised by uncertainty, fluidity and change. Positioning and reading the family, in these wider terms that are shifting and flexible, more centrally into our understanding of living with chronic conditions, we argue, is a way to make sense of, and indeed more purposefully manage, the ever-growing presence of chronic conditions in contemporary society.

## Self-care and management of chronic conditions: the place of the family?

There is little doubt that the management of long-term/chronic conditions is a major priority for health systems internationally: figures cited by the Department of Health (2012: 3) make this very clear.

> People with LTCs [long-term conditions] account for: 50% of all GP appointments; 64% of outpatient appointments; 70% of all inpatient bed days... in total around 70% of the total health and care spend in England (£7 out of every £10) is attributed to caring for people with LTCs. This means that 30% of the population account for 70% of the spend.

The social and economic pressure this places on health and social care services is evident and the predictions are that these costs are set to rise, particularly in the context of growing co-morbidities. In England, the number of people living with 'multiple LTCs is set to rise to 2.9 million in 2018 from 1.9 million in 2008' (Department of Health, 2012: 6). Indeed, multiple co-morbidities were a common feature for the overwhelming majority of people who participated in our study on living with lupus. These included lupus (most commonly) with Sjögren's disease, thyroid disease, Reynaud's syndrome and rheumatoid arthritis, among others. While the demographic context for the increase in chronic conditions is rightly assumed to be related to greater life expectancy, in the case of lupus and other autoimmune conditions, for example, age is certainly not always a factor and diagnosis in the mid, and sometimes early, life-course generates very particular vulnerabilities for those people and their families. This is a stage in life, of course, which is more generally neglected in research policy and the practice of healthcare, as it is often assumed to be a 'healthy', 'productive' and 'generative' stage.

Supporting people to live with chronic conditions has been a core focus of public health policy in the UK for well over a decade (Department of Health, 2001, 2005a, 2005b, 2008, 2009, 2010a, 2010b, 2012), and is based largely on 'system approaches used in the US such as the Kaiser Permanente "pyramid of care" and the Evercare model' (Hewison, 2012: 148). This policy context has been further consolidated, in, among other policy documents, the White Paper *Equity and Excellence: Liberating the NHS* (Department of Health, 2010a) and the Health and Social Care Act 2012 and the Care Act 2014 in which improved outcomes for people (and by definition the NHS) living with chronic, long-term conditions are central. A 'relentless focus on clinical outcomes' (Department of Health, 2010a: 1) and the 'patient in partnership with the health services' are the key underpinning principles of this policy framework – to be achieved through the goals of personalisation, choice, partnership working, shared decision making, and the use of new technologies (Department of Health, 2012: 18). The Department of Health (2012), for example, cites a number of positive examples of innovative approaches to care and services for people with chronic conditions. One case study of a 67-year-old woman living with fibromyalgia syndrome, osteoarthritis and Sjögren's syndrome, outlines how, with the use of a personal health budget, she has been able to secure help at home and funding to take up hobbies outside the house, all of which have positive health outcomes. There can be little doubt that self-management, self-care and patient empowerment is an important corrective to the biomedical tradition that is almost exclusively practitioner-led (Nettleton, 2013). The Expert Patient Programme (Department of Health, 2001) and personal health budgets are clear examples of programmes and indeed, as we have argued, ideological shifts that reflect patient empowerment and control. As Nicol (2011: 79) states: 'The aim of the EPP is, through self-management, to provide people, living with an LTC, with the knowledge, tools and skills to effectively manage their LTC and maintain control of their condition and life.' It is surprising, however, that family receives very little attention (or scrutiny) in this policy outcomes-based discourse. In the *Long Term Conditions Compendium of Information* (Department of Health, 2012), for example, there is quite simply no mention of family at all. The emphasis throughout is on the pursuit of improving individual health, largely devoid of the context within which health outcomes are realised. The individualisation of healthcare, self-care and self-management, at the expense of family or, indeed, community-based strategies for care and support, is, we would suggest, certainly a consequence of a personalised outcomes-based health and social care framework.

## Where is the family and how is the place (and nature) of the family considered in living with long-term conditions?

One place the family is to be found is in our reading and understanding of the concept of 'carers'.[1] Larkin (2012) suggests that the role of carers, now cemented in policy and legislation, is best understood in relation to the concept of community care.

The shift of healthcare from hospitals to the community (including family members) in the 1970s and 1980s in the UK provides the general context to formal 'caring', but, specifically, community care 'has come to be used to describe care for people in need which is based on support and care for individuals in their homes provided through a mixed economy of care' (Bytheway and Johnson, 1998; Larkin, 2012: 185). Informal care, the bedrock of community and largely gendered family relations, was formalised and legally enshrined in the NHS and Community Care Act (1990), which underpinned the statutory rights of carers as distinct and separate from those they 'cared for' – a critical semantic and legislative means of highlighting the potentially oppressive nature of 'relationships of obligation', thus dissolving a sense of 'family', and disaggregating the system that, until the new legislation, was a presumed feature of long-term conditions. This legislative framework has certainly functioned (more latterly) to recognise and protect both the cared and the cared for (certainly financially in terms of access to relevant funding) but has also served to fundamentally shape our understanding of care and caring in the family. That is, family relationships, have, in some respects, become formalised and legalised through policy guidance and legislation resulting in the fact that individual family members have effectively been 're-badged' as 'carers' or 'family caregivers' and the person diagnosed with a long-term condition, the 'cared for'. We understand, of course, that, as illness takes its toll and the basis for, and experience of, relationships change, this semantic shift may well be one that family members choose to operationalise themselves, that is, they self-identify as carers (for any number of reasons[2]) but the point remains that the process of re-badging family as 'carers' while recognising the supportive role that family play as carers, it also, perhaps, serves to obscure the ways in which this recasting might impact upon people's experiences and relationships. One of our questions, therefore, would be at what point does dependence and interdependence in relationships become 'care', funded or unfunded.

While, conceptually, this shift was very much needed at the time of the various reforms, Larkin (2012: 192) suggests that we need to look at the ways in which the modernisation agenda and its concomitant shift to personalised care has impacted on carers, which may lead 'to an erosion of a carer's self-identity and affect the dynamics of the relationship between people living with a long-term condition and their carer'. One result of this is that the voice of carers has become an increasingly prominent one in the context of patient empowerment more generally (Carr and Beresford, 2012). This voice has sought to articulate an identity and a place of authority. For example, during the course of our research, at a service user and carer conference[3] we attended in 2013, a mother of two children with autism argued that 'she was tired of being ignored and disregarded as their mother, she wanted a voice as their carer' – a voice that, ironically, wielded greater power and status, certainly in the health and social bureaucracies that she had to continually navigate. This semantic shift provided a critical identity for her and came with statutory rights and responsibilities. Intimate relationships are thus centrally implicated in sustaining and promoting self-care (for both 'carers' and 'cared for'). Arguably, this model of individualised patient empowerment and improved patient outcomes in the shift towards self-management rests on a fundamental assumption that relationships of intimacy within and between families and family members are medicalised. Lovers, partners, parents and siblings become facilitators of self-care in the pursuit of improved health and social care outcomes. This relationship between the notion of caring and that of family is, in our view, central to understanding how families view and manage chronic conditions. It is important to identify its complexity and move it beyond the traditional biomedical assumption of an assumed (welcome/necessary) shift. As one of our respondents, in the context of the relationship she shares with her husband, said to us:

> **Kerry:** He… gets fed up of caring, I think, or I don't know, he does get fed up, he doesn't like doing it, he doesn't like caring because he doesn't find that as part of his role. His role is my partner not, not my carer.

While the state may, therefore, have legislated family into the self-management of illness through the category of carer (which has undoubtedly had significant benefits for all parties in the caring relationship), the nature of 'caring' is complex, particularly in the context of an intimate relationship, where caring is about much more than individual health outcomes (see for example Richardson et al., 2007, who ask us to consider the idea of 'support' instead of 'care', both emotional and practical). Indeed, we were continually struck in the course of our research by the assumed replacement of, or slippage between, hitherto understood roles and identities of brother, partner, mother, husband and carer – at what point we wondered, did one begin and the other end? Nancy Mairs captures some of these complexities in her series of essays *Carnal Acts* (1990) about her life lived with multiple sclerosis. One of her reflections is on the nature of her 'caring' relationship with her husband, who she describes as a gifted caregiver. She says: 'He is just the sort of caregiver a fearful person needs: not a protector… but an encourager, one who gives heart for terrifying leaps into the unknown.' She speaks, perhaps, of a particular version of 'carer', somewhat removed from a medicalised understanding of the notion. Talking of a journey she made to Kinshasa to see her daughter (against the advice of the airline) she says:

> And this is the only way I know to live as a woman with multiple sclerosis: not to listen to the ominous questions of the Lufthansa agents but to hear instead the confidence (even if you think it is misplaced) of the daughter who believes that you're sure what you want to do, of the husband who says you can manage together…
>
> (Mairs, 1990: 161).

As we have noted, a medicalised and individualised understanding of the family and caring is one that is largely outcomes-based rather than relationship-focused, and questions of family processes and practices are often not foregrounded. In this context, for example, models and indicators of family support, which evaluate and measure family adaptation to illness and promote the best clinical outcomes, are identified (Knafl and Gilliss, 2002; Rosland and Piette, 2010; Rosland et al., 2012) and it is chronic disease management, in particular, which is often highlighted in the biomedical literature in this context (Lempp et al., 2006). While, importantly, the patient (and not the health practitioner) is central in this literature, the nature and subjective experience of the family/family relationships often does not come under the spotlight. Similarly, the psychological impact of living with chronic conditions is largely focused on individual coping strategies and the relationship, for example, between depression (and other mental health issues) and living with a chronic condition (Barlow, 2009). Gregory (2005) and Thompson et al. (2008) offer a different perspective and point to the importance of looking at family practices and family relationships in understanding chronic illness in a family setting, rather than the overtly one-dimensional framework outlined above. Thompson et al. (2008: 54) argue, for example: 'The impact of chronic illness on families has long been noted in the literature but in such studies families usually appear as ready-formed entities.' They go on to suggest that the work involved in the production of families, in the context of ill-health, is largely unacknowledged. It is the production of families in the context of managing and living with chronic conditions that is missing or is, at very least, opaque, in individualised, outcomes-based and medicalised accounts of coping.

The work of Gregory (2005) and Thompson et al. (2008) constitutes a critical thread in current debates within the sociology of family life that act as something of a rejoinder (and addition) to those conceptions outlined earlier, which most often present the family as a structured, reliable and somewhat inflexible entity (which is always present) that illness disrupts and unsettles (see for example the reviews by Knafl and Gilliss, 2002; Rosland and Piette, 2010; Rosland et al., 2012). Moreover, this framework often works on the assumption that families exist prior to illness, yet relationships will also inevitably be formed 'after illnesses' or during periods of (ongoing) uncertainty. That is, people living with chronic conditions will initiate and negotiate new relationships into which illness may be incorporated from the start. Static, taken for granted, formulations and those underpinning the policy/legislative context focus on the ways in which this previously stable form can be mobilised to support the ill person most effectively, helping to return the individual and, by definition, the family unit to its pre-illness state of equilibrium – assuming perhaps erroneously that there was an existing state of equilibrium. Their concern with the patient's individual experience of illness, neglects the wider impact on family relationships and thus misses the opportunity to reflect on the relationship between illness and families more generally (Denny and Earle, 2009; Meerabeau and Wright, 2011).

In contrast, we (in line with Gregory, 2005 and Thompson et al., 2008) suggest a rather different starting point – Morgan's (1996) 'influential idea of family practices in which the activities of families – the doing of family life [is] prioritised… over the construction of what a family is – who 'counts' as family' (Dermott and Seymour, 2011: 4). Morgan (2011: 3) sought to challenge concrete conceptions of 'the family' as if it had 'thing-like' qualities. In this way, he upset the idea that 'the family' had some kind of 'normative status', where normative, was nuclear, heterosexual, married with children: a conception that we know to be increasingly unreflective of contemporary British society, where blended and diverse family forms are increasingly 'normative' (Chambers, 2012). For example, Office of National Statistics (ONS) data indicate that, in the UK in 2012, there were 26.4 million households, of which 29 per cent consisted of only one person and almost 20 per cent consisted of four or more people. The idea of 'doing family', for Morgan (2011), was to shift our thinking from families as static structures. Rather, people within the family (family actors) are perceived to be 'doing parenting' and in the context of our explication of living in a family (or a relationship) with chronic illness, 'doing caring', for example. Morgan's (2011) conception of doing family in the context of family practices has prompted sociologists to understand the family in ways that have proved to be much more fluid, flexible and adaptable. Finch (2007, 2011) and others (in Dermott and Seymour, 2011) have extended this idea, suggesting that family must 'be displayed as well as done' and provide multiple empirical and theoretical case studies to this end. Finch (2007) defines 'display' as 'the process by which individuals, and groups of individuals, convey to each other and to relevant audiences that certain of their actions do constitute "doing family things" and thereby confirm that these relationships are "family" relationships' (Finch, 2011, cited in Dermott and Seymour, 2011: 4). In the contemporary context of multiple blended families, where the situation contests 'norms' of family and health, Finch (2007, 2011) argues that family practices have to be 'displayed', in order to secure acknowledgement and recognition.

There are two critical points that we would like to draw out of this discussion. The first is the reinsertion and application of a flexible conception of the family to biomedical traditions that render it unbending. People living with chronic illness draw on family relationships that are multiple and varied – an understanding that is crucial in the context of autoimmune conditions, which may themselves be particularly complex and uncertain. The family (and its relationships) is unpredictable, inherently variable, blended and shifting. We suggest that there are clear and helpful parallels to be drawn between a flexible understanding of family and family relationships and illnesses that belie a linear trajectory model (of symptoms, diagnosis, treatment, cure or long-term disability and death). The second point is the notion of 'display'. We suggest that the coupling of illness and display, within the broad rubric of 'displaying family', illuminates the ways in which people convey their distress, pain, understanding, support, needs and desires to one another and the health professionals with which they are interacting. Illness becomes an additional display and dimension of family experience that is variously negotiated and that comes to constitute a further layer and dimension of family practice – of doing and displaying family. We can then capture, as Chesla (2005: 373) suggests, some of the paradoxes of living with chronic illness where families 'live with days of intense suffering, small suffering, and chronic depression, mixed with moments of delight and possibility. They live lives filled with both.'

How, then, does living a life with an unpredictable, shifting condition take place within the family? How, and in what ways, does it change and mediate relationships, expectations, roles and identities? How, in particular, does it intersect with the issues of gender and parenting? How do people negotiate their changing normalities and how does the practice and experience of caring change in the context of intimate relationships? In our own work, these questions were central to our exploration of illness in the context of family and, indeed, of family in the context of illness. The gendered and corporeal effects of lupus on the family (specifically its doing and production) were highlighted repeatedly in the interviews we undertook. Intimacy, partnership and motherhood, in particular, were resonant themes that suggested to us that relationships with partners and the nature of those partnerships require extensive renegotiation when a chronic condition becomes a feature of family life. Doing family in this context can be very challenging, not least because the care and support provided is very much embodied, involving emotional and intimate engagement with the body in which ways which are often unfamiliar (Morgan, 2011; Parker and Seymour, 1998). Capturing the complexity (clinical necessity, embarrassment and intimacy) of this bodywork (Twigg, 2006), Irene said:

> I had the pain in my joints, in my muscles, I couldn't move, I couldn't get off the bed and my husband rang the doctor and said, well I can't bring her in because she can't move off the bed. So then he had to try and get a specimen of urine off me and my husband had to try somehow and get this specimen and it was really like blood.

The bodily living and doing of chronic conditions challenge and reconfigure everyday intimacies. Bodies, sites of shared pleasure, also become everyday and often mundane sites of illness and shared distress. The participants in our study spoke, for example, of the 'public'/family difficulties of dealing with mouth and nose ulcers, dry mouths, rashes, diarrhoea, vomiting, acid reflux and weight gain.

> **Lucy:** I went from six stone five to nine stone ten and it was like a big ring all around my stomach and when I sat down I had this big ring round my stomach and the doctor kept on to me, oh what are you worried about your weight for? I said, it is not so much my weight, I said my stomach is sitting on my legs when I sit down and I've just got this great big ring and if I eat anything, by the time night-time comes I'm in so much discomfort I can't sit down because my stomach is so bloated.

Our data suggests that illness not only calls into question the nature of embodied care, but also unsettles the doing of gender in the family. Andrew pointed to the ways in which he felt unable to perform masculinity either as a husband, father or grandfather.

> **Andrew:** Instead of me looking after mine, mine are looking after me and that isn't the way round I want it to be, you know... it sort of takes away your masculinity really... you feel weak, you feel a feeling of inadequacy.

In this same context, some of the women we interviewed expressed anxiety at not being able to perform tasks traditionally associated with women in the home, while their partners assumed many of their traditional gendered roles and tasks in the family context.

> **Alan:** To me personally, [illness] mostly probably brought the woman part out of me, and I don't mean [laughs] I don't know how to switch on the washing

machine or the dishwasher or the hoover… but the things I can do to help her, I do all the cooking now, because… I feel that it's a risk if she goes near because… she's got… the arthritis and rheumatism part of it and that, so I will do that, so that relieves her of one duty.

Indeed, rebalancing and renegotiating traditional gender roles are an ongoing feature of family life in the context of chronic conditions. In her study of family practices in diet related chronic illness, Gregory (2005) found that family (gendered) identities and expectations did not necessarily shift as a result of illness, rather, she argues, traditional gender roles (in the face of illness), while more porous and malleable than expected, nonetheless remain firm. 'Within the family, well or ill, members are also mother, father, spouse, child, but these identities do not always allow for concessions to be made for illness' (Gregory, 2005: 381). Similarly, Townsend et al. (2014), in a study of women's accounts of help-seeking in early rheumatoid arthritis, also point to men's and women's determination to maintain family/gender roles and responsibilities. In an effort to maintain parenting responsibilities, one woman said for example, 'I could barely walk. I would hobble along… I was a homemaker at the time so… I used to push myself … when the kids were young I would stay up really late to clean the house. And even if I was tired I would say: "No I'm going to keep doing this"' (Townsend et al., 2014: 5). As was the case with our research, Lempp et al. (2006), in a study of the impact of rheumatoid arthritis on personal identity, point to a discernible shift in gender roles in the home, 'Everybody helps out, I don't have a choice. I don't think my kids miss out; my little one may be, because I can't go out with her, swimming for example. But my sister and husband and other family members take them out. My husband does a lot of the housework now. He does work hard to keep things going' (Lempp et al., 2006: 112).

The adjustments people made to their family lives and the negotiations they engaged in in order to accommodate and resist the effects of illness also became part and parcel of day-to-day life for many of our own respondents.

> **Alan:** We've been married a long time, so, you know, it's not a case of 'oh, I've had enough of this' and walked out. You do have your blips and think, 'Oh God, I've got to do this again', but you just get over it. I've come to understand it and once you start to understand it and know the pain that your partner is going through then you just adjust your life.

This couple's son was in New York when we interviewed them and he was sending back pictures of his adventures there, which included skating on an open air ice rink. Harriet took up the conversation and said, 'I would love to go on that' but Alan interrupted:

> I'd love to take her, but unless we can get something from the doctor saying, right, you're guaranteed to be okay, you're not going to have any embolisms or anything, you just can't take the chance and I cannot afford to lose her.

The display of love and affection here is clearly mediated through illness for this couple. Incorporating illness into their relationship involved not just a readjustment of displays of care but also focused on the necessity to 'reset normal' family life, such that illness shaped where they could and could not go and how they conducted their days. Adjusting to fear, anxiety and loss in the context of family relationships was a recurring theme throughout our interviews, where the common refrain was, 'you can still get on with your life, you have to still get on with your life'. Some of the women in Barker's (2005) study of fibromyalgia, spoke similarly of family adjustment and absorption:

> Fibromyalgia affects how you feel about yourself. Your family sees this person that used to be able to do everything, who all of a sudden you can't even prepare a meal. You have to work through all this emotional stuff. You have no self-esteem but you have to find a way to go on.
>
> (Barker, 2005: 86)

In a study of family relationships in supporting self-care in an online environment, Sanders et al. (2011) identify the importance of online support for people living with chronic conditions, in large part because of the pressures that managing illness places on family relationships. In this study, participants pointed to the challenges of adjusting to illness. One participant said, 'Does anyone else get snappy and irritable with loved ones?' (Sanders et al., 2011: 141). Another said, 'I too become evil with my family especially my husband. With me though it isn't just pain it is such total frustration with myself and inability to cope. It is dreadful because I too love them all dearly.' Yet, the authors point to the demands and challenges participants face in an attempt to live a 'normal and successful life': a woman living with rheumatoid arthritis said, 'I think we nearly kill ourselves trying to continue as normal because we don't want to give in' (Sanders et al., 2011: 142).

In an earlier study, Thompson et al. (2008: 193) speak of the 'moral work' involved in managing multiple chronic conditions. In their study, participants 'spoke of their desire to act as one "should" in the face of debilitating symptoms. For example... [performing] domestic tasks as "a mother"'. Ironically, in the context of the discussion earlier in this chapter, the 'moral imperative' to 'keep going' is at odds, they argue, with the fundamental principles of self-care/management – keeping the family going was not best for their physical health.

For many families (and couples) in our study, living with illness was something that had characterised their relationship from the outset (often because diagnosis took place over many years). As such, their encounter with illness, and the ways in which it was mediated in the context of their relationships, constituted a series of ongoing, lifelong adjustments. In a joint interview with her husband, Victoria (now in her late 50s) said:

> You went with me for my first x-ray when I was 17 because we knew then that there was something wrong, so I suppose you should have really kicked me into touch years ago, but here you are, nearly 40 years later.

The dynamics of intimacy and partnering between and within families living with chronic conditions are continually reset and renegotiated at different points on the illness journey and we have pointed to the gendered nature of some of these shifts. Mothering and motherhood is a further dimension of this. Our participants spoke throughout of the challenges of adjusting motherhood to illness and illness to motherhood.

Becoming a mother is sometimes extremely difficult for women living with lupus. A number of women who participated in our study spoke of their distress at having experienced a miscarriage (miscarriage sometimes constituted part of the diagnostic process). Debbie who has lupus and Hughes' syndrome (also known as antiphospholipid syndrome, a lupus-related condition in which there is an increased tendency to blood clotting) said:

> My late 20s and early 30s were plagued by a series of miscarriages. I had two miscarriages at 10–12 weeks, then twins at a later stage. Since I was moving around the country, no one made the connection between Hughes' and miscarriage. It wasn't until 1998 when I had my first and only child that there seemed to be a plummet into ill health. Having had a very difficult pregnancy – placenta praevia grade 4, ++++ protein and anaemia – my son was eight weeks premature and very poorly, as was I. I was in intensive care for two days due to large blood loss and my boy was in SCBU for a month. Almost immediately after the birth I became ill, plagued with joint pain, blisters on the skin, ear, sinus infections, migraine and a despairing depression. Then in 2003 I had a stroke. I was a high school teacher and it happened in a lesson, I felt like I had been hit with a baseball bat!

As we have previously outlined, some people, the decision to have children was also very much shaped by their condition/s.

> **Lydia:** The prospect of having children is a big part of my life. I did not want to be a young mum but now I find myself thinking, how long do I wait? What happens if in five years' time I am not well enough to have children or will I even be able to? I am on methotrexate and I know that I am not allowed to conceive on these tablets and they have helped me so much so the thought of having to give up those tablets scares me. Also, my consultant has said not to even think of children right now.

> **Shireen:** I am told I cannot try for a baby now as the lupus is still active, but I am desperate to try. I was told the same thing one year ago. It is so frustrating, I am 30 years old and healthy, apart from the lupus and it is now stopping me from starting a family.

For women with children, it was their fear and the need to conceal and offset it for the benefit of others that generated much additional anxiety.

> **Molly:** I can feel she's [daughter] watching me all the time and she'll say, are you alright? And you'll think I feel fine, do I look tired? Am I tired? And I wish she

wouldn't say it but I think she is so frightened of something happening that she watches me all the time and, you know, I can feel her.

**Lucy:** I don't like whinging, about it. My children get so easily panicked.

The struggle to mother, to protect children and to keep the family functioning at all costs (see Townsend et al., 2014) in face of long-term illness was extremely difficult, yet generative at times.

> **Irene:** Sometimes in my bed I'm thinking I don't want to live like this, I want to die, but then pop, that thought goes because I think what about your children, what about the children? And then I used to pray, please God just let me live that my children are older and can fend for themselves because I know they couldn't depend on their dad… So I prayed for that and then I feel that's been given to me and then I've got beautiful grandchildren.

Edwards (2013: 6), writing 'as a lifelong patient with multiple illnesses', speaks of her need to display good, loving motherhood in spite of her illnesses. She says: 'Every day, I wake up, feed my child, take my medications, and put on the trappings of the well. I am her mother, first and foremost, and that does not change depending on my symptoms.' She continues (after also describing her continued commitment to work/teaching), 'I am used to such deceiving appearances, and I depend on technology to keep up the facade when I need it' (Edwards, 2013: 6). Invoking Sontag's (2001) metaphor of the movement between the kingdom of the sick and the kingdom of the well, Edwards (2013: 6) says: 'I am not alone in this daily negotiation, and beyond the numbers are the compromises and compensations made by all people living with some form of chronic condition.' Kathlyn Conway's journal that documents her struggle with three cancers is a poignant account of how hard it is to be a mother in this context. She says: 'When Molly and Zach return from school I struggle fairly unsuccessfully to be a good mother. I try to listen to Molly's piano practicing, but I am completely distracted. Zach tells me about his homework assignments, but I can barely comprehend what he is saying' (Conway, 2007: 142).

Ongoing daily struggles with illness similarly left some mothers in our study battling with feelings of inadequacy and guilt.

> **Irene:** I couldn't help my children, because I had this pain so badly, and I felt useless. I felt I am no good for, to my children and you know, not so long ago, about last year I heard my daughter talking to a friend and she says well, you know, you were lucky because I didn't have my mum to go shopping and I didn't have my mum to go about, because she was [ill]. She said I didn't have my mum since I was nine. I didn't have my mum, so you are very lucky.

Accepting help and support from their children also left both men and women in our study feeling conflicted.

**Lucy:** My children have been so good, they've supported me, they've sat and cried with me when I've cried, they've sat on the bed, they've bathed me when I can't even get out of bed to have a bath and that, you know, and, and they've been absolutely fantastic, you know, so I've been really lucky. But, because it got to the point where it was upsetting them so much I didn't tell them, unless I needed their help and I'd ring and say not too good today, could you do some shopping?

Nicki, whose husband worked away during the week talked about the help her son (12 years old) gave her:

He'll empty the dishwasher and you know, all that sort of stuff, just, 'you sit down Mummy, I'll make you a cup of tea'… bless him.

In the context of chronic illness, being a mother and being mothered extends, reverses and cements the boundaries and expectations of family relationships. A woman living with chronic fatigue syndrome, whose experiences are documented by Edwards (2013: 103), says: 'It's hard to be a grown woman and depend on your mother for a place to live, food to eat, the ability to take a shower or get to a doctor's appointment.' In an essay on living with rheumatoid arthritis, Vervaecke (1998) poignantly sums up this complex cycle of inter/dependence. She is writing about going home (to her mother) with her young son, describing her exhaustion, the smells, textures and memories of home. She is, however, unable to bathe her son due to her inability to use her hands. The simple pleasures of bath-time are, she states, reserved for her more able mother, rather than herself. It is, however, a solace for her that it is her mother who is performing the mundane (integral to everyday life), tasks that her illness intrudes upon.

Through the lens of intimacy and motherhood, then, we have looked at some of the ways in which chronic conditions change and mediate family practices and particularly at how long-term conditions intersect with the 'doing' and 'displaying' of gender and parenting. In extending Morgan's (1996, 2011) concept of 'family as a process rather than an entity', Gregory (2005: 388) argues that the term 'family relationship suggests a processual acting out of everyday, sometimes mundane, domestic tasks and activities that constitute individual and family identities, through understandings of "the normal family life"'. Gregory suggests that the pursuit of 'normality' – routine and repeated family practices – in the context of chronic illness offers ontological security. In her study, gender was a negotiated but enduring medium through which family/illness relationships played themselves out and thus 'the participants in [her] study accommodated the intrusion of chronic illness by relying upon an understanding of both personal and family identities for which gender was just one (important) factor' (Gregory, 2005: 389). Family practices, Gregory (2005: 389–390) suggests, can be both 'predictable and stable, while encompassing change and uncertainty'. With this understanding, families could then adjust (including adjustments of intimacies and gender relations) to new constraints which long-term illness demands while retaining a sense of 'ontological security' – they could 'construct and lead a normal life'. Drawing on Sanderson et al.'s (2011) model of 'normalities' we discussed in Chapter 4, we suggest that the security and normality to which Gregory refers is, however, continually shifting in the context of many autoimmune conditions (where symptoms can change on a daily basis) – lupus (and evidentially rheumatoid arthritis, scleroderma, multiple sclerosis, etc.) continually impose 'new normals' on individuals and families – which generate their own particular 'ontological (in)securities'. This demands particular forms of family practice that require the most exquisitely sensitive accommodation on the illness journey from all concerned. As Sharon said of her partner:

> I've been really, really lucky in that he's understood and as I've moved through my illness, he has moved with me.

## Families living and doing illness

In this chapter we argue that placing the patient at the centre of their care – in the social context of their families, networks (Vassilev et al., 2011) and other significant relationships – is arguably one of the most appropriate ways of optimising health/clinical outcomes. Conceptually, as well as practically, it is vital to explicitly locate the family within the conception and management of long-term conditions. It is both short-sighted and inadequate to assume or take its presence for granted. Conceiving of the individual (and by association their family and support network) largely in terms of linear outcome-based models of (cost-)effectiveness is, we would argue, a missed opportunity to understand and respond to the everyday challenges of living with a chronic health condition. A model of self-care that accommodates flexibility and uncertainty is perhaps at odds with a one-dimensional model which focuses only on clinical outcomes, yet a dynamic understanding of family practices is arguably a more nuanced way to respond to the everyday, ever-changing demands of being a mother, a partner, a parent, a child, a sibling or a lover living with one or multiple chronic health conditions. In this way, it may be the case that health practitioners can save lives and relationships even if they can't cure the patient.

What then is the place of social work in achieving this? As we have argued, the family constitutes a critical medium through which chronic illness is lived, yet it also lies at the heart of social work practice – for social work/ers the family is an essential social institution and a primary reference point. The family is regarded as a source of, and place for, care, respite and generativity. It is a central point of support and intimacy and provides a reservoir of resource and resilience (as we know, of course, it is also a place of potential harm and risk). The family very often constitutes the starting point for an assessment of state support and social work intervention. It is the basis upon which services are organised and are either forthcoming or not. The place of social work in supporting illness and its resulting vulnerability in the family is, however, less clear and is arguably largely ignored in both social work practice and the relevant literature. It is this neglect in what is a critical space for nurture and intervention that constitutes the focus of our final chapter

# Notes

1 We are following Larkin's definition of carer. She says the term carer is 'used to refer to someone caring for a person who cannot care for him/herself and, excluding benefits, carries this out on an unpaid basis' (Larkin, 2012: 185).
2 This might most obviously pertain, for example, in situations where a person's condition might be seen to alter them (and thus the ways they are able to relate to others). We have, in mind, the debate as it relates to people living with dementia and other cognitive challenges.
3 Service User Carer Group Conference, University of Hull, 16 July 2013.

# References

Barker, K. K. (2005) *The Fibromyalgia Story: Medical Authority and Women's Worlds of Pain.* Philadelphia: Temple University Press.

Barlow, J. (2009) *Living with Arthritis.* West Sussex: BPS Blackwell.

Beresford, P. (2014) *Personalisation.* Bristol: Policy Press.

Bytheway, B. and Johnson, J. (1998) 'The Social Construction of "Carers"'. In A. Symonds and A. Kelly (eds), *The Social Construction of Community Care.* London: Macmillan.

CarersUK Online (no date) www.carersuk.org (accessed 20 June 2014).

Carers (Equal Opportunities) Act 2004, www.legislation.gov.uk/ukpga/2004/15/pdfs/ukpga_20040015_en.pdf (accessed 20 June 2014).

Carers Recognition and Services Act 1995, www.legislation.gov.uk/ukpga/1995/12/pdfs/ukpga_19950012_en.pdf (accessed 20 June 2014).

Carr, S. and Beresford, P. (2012) *Social Care, Service Users and User Involvement.* London: Jessica Kingsley Publishers.

Chambers, D. (2012) *A Sociology of Family Life: Change and Diversity in Intimate Relations.* Cambridge: Polity Press.

Chesla, C. A. (2005) 'Nursing Science and Chronic Illness: Articulating Suffering and Possibility in Family Life'. *Journal of Family Nursing* 11(4): 371–387.

Conway, K. (2007) *Ordinary Life: A Memoir of Illness.* Michigan: University of Michigan Press.

Denny, E. and Earle, S. (2009) *The Sociology of Long Term Conditions and Nursing Practice.* London: Palgrave Macmillan.

Department of Health (2001) *The Expert Patient: A New Approach to Chronic Disease Management in the 21st Century.* London: The Stationery Office.

Department of Health (2005a) *Supporting People with Long-Term Conditions: An NHS and Social Care Model to Support Local Innovation and Integration.* London: HMSO.

Department of Health (2005b) *National Service Framework for Long-Term Conditions.* London: Department of Health.

Department of Health (2006) *Our Health, Our Care, Our Say.* London: HMSO.

Department of Health (2007) *Putting People First: A Shared Vision and Committment to the Transformation of Adult Social Care,* http://webarchive.nationalarchives.gov.uk/20130107105354/www.dh.gov.uk/en/Publicationsandstatistics/Publications/PublicationsPolicyAndGuidance/DH_081118 (accessed 22 May 2014).

Department of Health (2008) *Your Health, Your Way: A Guide to Long-Term Conditions and Self Care.* London: Department of Health.

Department of Health (2009) *Supporting People with Long-term Conditions – Commissioning Personalised Care Planning.* London: Department of Health.

Department of Health (2010a) *Equity and Excellence: Liberating the NHS.* London: Department of Health.

Department of Health (2010b) *Improving the Health and Well-being of People with Long-term Conditions: World Class Services for People with Long-term Conditions – Information Tool for Big Commissioners*. London: Department of Health.

Department of Health (2012) *Long Term Conditions Compendium of Information*, www.gov.uk/ government/uploads/system/uploads/attachment_data/file/216528/dh_134486.pdf (accessed 22 May 2014).

Dermott, E. and Seymour, J. (2011) 'Developing "Displaying Families": A Possibility for the Future of the Sociology of Personal Life'. In E. Dermott and J. Seymour (eds), *Displaying Families: A New Concept for the Sociology of Family Life*. Basingstoke: Palgrave Macmillan.

Edwards, L. (2013) *In the Kingdom of the Sick: A Social History of Chronic Illness in America*. New York: Walker Publishing Company.

Finch, J. (2007) 'Displaying Families'. *Sociology* 41: 65–81.

Finch, J. (2011) 'Exploring the Concept of Display in Family Relationships'. In E. Dermott and J. Seymour (eds), *Displaying Families: A New Concept for the Sociology of Family Life*. Basingstoke: Palgrave Macmillan.

Gregory, S. (2005) 'Living with Chronic Illness in the Family Setting'. *Sociology of Health & Illness* 27(3): 372–392.

Hewison, A. (2012) 'Delivering Health and Social Care for People with Long-term Conditions: The Policy Context'. In C. E. Lloyd and T. Heller (eds), *Long-Term Conditions: Challenges in Health & Social Care*. London: Sage.

Knafl, K. A. and Gilliss, C. L. (2002) 'Families and Chronic Illness: A Synthesis of Current Research'. *Journal of Family Nursing* 8(3): 178–198.

Larkin, M. (2012) 'What About the Carers?' In C.E. Lloyd and T. Heller (eds), *Long-Term Conditions: Challenges in Health & Social Care*. London: Sage.

Lempp, H., Scott, D. and Kingsley, G. (2006) 'The Personal Impact of Rheumatoid Arthritis on Patients' Identity: A Qualitative Study'. *Chronic Illness* 2: 109–120.

Mairs, N. (1990) *Carnal Acts*. New York: HarperCollins.

Meerabeau, L. and Wright, K. (2011) *Long-Term Conditions: Nursing Care and Management*. London: Wiley-Blackwell.

Morgan, D. H. J. (1996) *Family Connections: An Introduction to Family Studies*. Cambridge: Polity Press.

Morgan, D. H. J. (2011) *Rethinking Family Practices*. Basingstoke: Palgrave Macmillan.

National Health Service and Community Care Act 1990, www.legislation.gov.uk/ ukpga/1990/19/contents (accessed 22 May 2014).

Nettleton, S. (2013) *Sociology of Health and Illness*, 3rd edition. Cambridge: Polity Press.

Nicol, J. (2011) *Nursing Adults with Long Term Conditions*. London: Sage.

Office for National Statistics (2012) *Families and Households 2012*, www.ons.gov.uk/ons/ dcp171778_284823.pdf (accessed 18 June 2014).

Parker, G. and Seymour, J. (1998) 'Male Carers in Marriage: Re-examining Feminist Analysis of Informal Care'. In J. Popay., J. Hearn and J. Edwards (eds), *Men, Gender Divisions and Welfare*. London: Routledge.

Richardson, J. C., Ong, B. N. and Sim, J. (2007) 'Experiencing Chronic Widespread Pain in a Family Context: Giving and Receiving Practical and Emotional Support'. *The Sociology of Health & Illness* 29(3): 347–365.

Rosland, A. and Piette, J. D. (2010) 'Emerging Models for Mobilizing Family Support for Chronic Disease Management: A Structured Review'. *Chronic Illness* 6: 7–21.

Rosland, A., Heisler, M. and Piette, J.D. (2012) 'The Impact of Family Behaviours and Communication Patterns on Chronic Outcomes: A Systematic Review'. *Journal of Behavioural Medicine* 35: 221–239.

Sanders, C., Rogers, A., Gardner, C. and Kennedy, A. (2011) 'Managing "Difficult Emotions" and Family Life: Exploring Insights and Social Support Within Online Self-management Training'. *Chronic Illness* 7(2): 134–146.

Sanderson, T., Calnan, M., Morris, M., Richards, P. and Hewlett, S. (2011) 'Shifting Normalities: Interactions of Changing Conceptions of a Normal Life and the Normalisation of Symptoms in Rheumatoid Arthritis'. *Sociology of Health & Illness* 33(4): 618–633.

Sontag, S. (2001) *Illness as Metaphor and AIDS and its Metaphors*. London: Picador.

Thompson, D., Thomas, H., Solomons, J., Nashef, L. and Kendall, S. (2008) 'Chronic Illness, Reproductive Health and Moral Work: Women's Experiences of Epilepsy'. *Chronic Illness* 4: 54–64.

Townsend, A., Backman, C. L., Adam, P. and Li, L. C. (2014) 'Women's Accounts of Help-seeking in Early Rheumatoid Arthritis from Symptom Onset to Diagnosis'. *Chronic Illness*.

Twigg, J. (2006) *The Body in Health and Social Care*. Basingstoke: Palgrave Macmillan.

Twigg, J. and Atkin, C. (1994) *Carers Perceived: Policy and Practice in Informal Care*. Buckingham: Open University Press.

Vassilev, I., Rogers, A., Sanders, C., Kennedy, A., Blickem, C., Protherroe, J., Bower, P., Kirk, S., Chew-Graham, C. and Morris, R. (2011) 'Social Networks, Social Capital and Chronic Illness Self-management: A Realist Review'. *Chronic Illness* 7: 60–68.

Vervaecke, K. (1998) 'Back in the Body'. In P. Foster and M. Swander (eds), *The Healing Circle*. New York: Plume.

# 8   Body work in social work

I've never thought, I've never thought of it [social work], in the need for physical illness. I've only seen social workers for families that can't cope.

(Myf)

Without exception, the respondents in our study, as the quote above indicates, had never encountered or even thought of drawing on the skills of a social worker in the course of being diagnosed or living with their illness. In a context where, as social workers, every aspect of our (professional) lives is embodied, this is deeply ironic but not unsurprising for, on the one hand, bodies are integral to social work practice, for social work (certainly within a statutory context) is in the business of observing, managing, policing, legislating for, resourcing and organising the care of bodies, controlling largely 'disenfranchised [and unhealthy] bodies' (Tangenberg and Kemp, 2002: 9). Yet, never has the physical body been more distant: social work's relationship with the physical body seems, at best, ambiguous and, at worst, unseen and perceived as irrelevant.

This chapter is centred on the questions foregrounded by this paradox: we ask what is the relationship of social work to the body and how do we account for the invisibility of corporeality in the profession? Here we aim to assert the importance and role of the physical body in social work practice and focus, in particular, on the ways in which physical health, illness and well-being should be appropriately incorporated, not only at either end of the life course, which is most often the case in social work practice. Indeed, it is the mundane everyday embodied weariness, the inexplicable and debilitating fatigue, 'the small sufferings', the confusing and arbitrary symptoms that continually shift and move throughout the body (Miles, 2014; Sanderson et al., 2011) – that is the reality of a life lived with chronicity, which, we suggest, should be central to an embodied, corporeal social work practice: a practice that embraces both the vulnerability generated by ill-health and the ill-health exacerbated by vulnerability. Drawing on the insights of the respondents interviewed in our study, we aim to offer a practice perspective that integrates medical knowledge and subjective experience, thus potentially claiming/reclaiming the territory of 'body work', which social work has, we would argue, abdicated to medicine and other health professionals (Twigg et al., 2011).

## Accounting for the invisibility of the physical body: the policy context

One explanation for the abdication we refer to may lie within the broader ideological and policy context within which social work has operated for the past 25 years and, among other things, the structural changes this has engendered. Throughout the 1980s, a neoliberal administration in the UK reconceptualised and reorganised public services to reflect the political will to decentralise and, arguably, destabilise centrally organised and provided welfare. The NHS and Community Care Act (1990) (NHSCCA) was, perhaps, emblematic of this political sea change and it assumed a pivotal place in the conceptualisation and subsequent reorganisation of the social work profession. This Act reflected an ideology that proposed radically new ways of working, including major structural changes to the delivery of social services, wherein many local authorities split their children's and adult provision (Lymbery, 2001; McLaughlin, 2009; Postle, 2001). The resulting mixed economy of care, with its central bureaucratic system of service brokerage, was a practice context in which 'recipients of care became customers and social workers practicing with adults were re-designated as care managers. This new name reflects a changed role as well as the generally enhanced importance of management and managers since the 1980s' (Harlow, 2003: 30). The explicit political objective embedded in these changes was the ostensibly altruistic aim of increasing choice, quality and availability of services, while decreasing bureaucracy and state interference. In reality, these changes were implicitly intended to simply reduce public expenditure (Harlow et al., 2013; Postle, 2001). This ideology is perhaps best exemplified by the ways in which the Thatcher administration planned the systematic closure of many of the UK's large psychiatric institutions without adequate funding or planning for the future care needs of this population of service users. This resulted in a moral panic and a situation in which ex-psychiatric in-patients were effectively made homeless without recourse to effective or timely community-based services (Foster and Roberts, 1999; Killaspy, 2006). In this new era, the context of social work provision, perhaps most easily identifiable in work with vulnerable adults (Harlow et al., 2013), was one in which it was not necessarily essential to be a qualified social worker to procure, broker and evaluate service provision – an effective route to the deprofessionalisation of social work more broadly (Dominelli, 1996).

The resulting shift in the ways in which social workers operated, which was underpinned by a commitment to new managerialism and technicism, both in the context of team-working and in the relationships shared with the new consumers of care, meant a move away from the traditional relationships that social workers and service users had previously shared. Social work tasks were now provided at a distance, further removing professionals from the physical interface with service users. This sense of distance was underpinned by the split between the commission/procurement and actual provision of services, a spilt that effectively separated out the range of tasks historically undertaken by social workers. This fragmentation 'redefined the role of social services from that of assessor and provider of services to that of "enabler", "commissioner" or "purchaser"' (McLaughlin, 2009: 1104). In this context of fragmentation and deprofessionalisation, social workers became care mangers and clients became consumers, customers, users and purchasers of social work services (McLaughlin, 2009). Harlow et al. (2013) go on to note that the profession became increasingly technicist, with social workers focusing on the component competencies of social work practice (the reception, assessment, intervention and review of service provision) rather than the interpersonal aspects of intervention. The managerial technicist practice is, therefore, concerned with what is observable and measurable at the expense of the use of the social worker's self. That is: 'The managerial context that emphasises rationality, fragmentation, technicism, and positivistic evaluation of performance, denies the emotional context of practice and the significance of relationship' (Harlow, 2003: 38). What, arguably, underpinned and shored up the move to technicist practice and a reduction in public expenditure was a focus on the initial assessment and screening (out) of need, which involved non-qualified workers making critical decisions about the trajectory of enquires into statutory social work teams. This meant that social workers were less visible and, critically, less accessible in the context of decision-making and potential intervention (Lymbery, 2001).

This destabilisation of a key component of the welfare continuum, it has been argued, was at the heart of Margaret Thatcher's aim to withdraw the state from the provision of welfare services. A direct consequence of this was the growth of the voluntary/private welfare sector at the expense of state provision (Lymbery, 2001). The roles that stayed firmly within the purview of professional social work, of course, were those concerning child protection and corporate parenting (Harlow, 2013). Adult social work assumed a less central, and arguably less important, position in the lexicon of professional, statutory, social work practice.

In the context of adult social work in particular, the changes noted above were occurring in a significant period of demographic shift, in which the older population was growing alongside the attendant requirements for long-term support (without a concomitant financial commitment to provide for it). More broadly, changes in the UK economy meant that service users across age groups were experiencing increased levels of poverty and deprivation, as Lymbery (2001: 373) notes, 'the degree of poverty endured by people in receipt of social services increased thereby exacerbating a range of other social problems'. In practice, this meant that statutory social work intervention became increasingly focused on immediate crisis response and intervention to the neglect of preventative social work. The widening gap between needs and resources was the social and political backdrop to these fundamental and ongoing changes in professional social work.

A change in government in 1997 did little to change the ideological underpinnings of welfare provision in the UK, despite ushering in further significant changes to the ways in which welfare services for adults were provided and received. Under the broad rubric of 'modernisation', represented as necessary to protect and enhance the services and safety of service users/clients/patients, business and managerial solutions to social problems and matters of social policy prevailed – sharpening accountability on the one hand and generating a culture of performance targets, inspection and auditing on the other; further constricting the place and role of adult social workers. New Labour's programme of welfare reform thus continued the increasingly firmly established themes of individualisation, responsibilisation and the privatisation of risk (Ferguson, 2007). The introduction of Direct Payments in 1996, initially under the Conservative government (Community Care (Direct Payments) Act 1996), was without doubt (and remains) the most significant development in adult social care to date. Direct Payments allowed local authorities to provide cash in lieu of services, thus enabling individuals to buy their own care (McLaughlin, 2009), unquestionably providing a vehicle that facilitated the transfer of power from those who provide services to those who use them. However, people requiring social work support and intervention are not always in a position to manage, control and shape their 'care packages' and the role of social workers (in the provision of statutory services) remains circumscribed and curtailed, as does the visibility and place of the physical body within social work practice; a further irony, given the original convergence of Direct Payments with the disability rights movement's aim for greater individual control over support needs (Glendinning et al., 2000).

The notion of personalisation, subsequent to and incorporating Direct Payments (and more latterly personal budgets), remains at the heart of government policy on adult social care (Department of Health, 2005; 2008; 2010; 2012) and impacts directly, if ambiguously, on contemporary social work practice (Ferguson, 2007). Lymbery (2012) suggests that, at first glance, the ideology of personalisation fits comfortably with the core elements of social work (social change, social well-being, human rights and social justice); however, he cautions that narrow interpretations that focus on individual need, to the exclusion of social need, restrict the wider 'empowering' possibilities of personalisation. Indeed, Ferguson (2007) argues that the individual experience of health and social care cannot be separated from structural inequities – the production of health and welfare services (in, for example, the machinations of personalisation) play only a relatively small part in the production and maintenance of people's health and well-being. It is the structural context, not simply that of individual empowerment, which arguably requires attention, for it is the social determinants of health that most profoundly influence health outcomes. Health and social care services and interventions account for only 20 per cent of our health status – the far greater balance (80 per cent) is overwhelmingly determined by life chances, including, for example, education, early childhood intervention and employment with payment at the living wage (British Academy, 2014; Marmot Review, 2010).

While personalisation can be seen as a mechanism for restoring and championing people's rights, it is also the case that the realisation of choice is not an entirely rational process. As Lymbery (2012: 788) argues, 'if we take into account the physical and cognitive frailties of many people in need of services, there are apparent limitations on their ability both to exercise choice and to have that choice turned into positive action'. The social, physical and cultural capital required to design, procure and manage services and sources of care cannot be underestimated. These contradictions that sit at the heart of personalisation are rendered more complex in a context of financial austerity and severe cost-cutting that has taken place, and continues to take place, within social care, situating the poorest in society at greater risk. Moreover, the rapidly expanding care needs of an ageing population will inevitably place further demands on shrinking services. Lymbery (2012) points to the impact this has on prevention and early intervention strategies and the restrictions (and constrictions) of ever tightening eligibility threshold criteria: 'The potential of social work to offer a proactive and positive supporting role within the framework of personalisation is therefore being severely constrained' (Lymbery, 2012: 789). The transformational possibilities offered by personalisation, personal budgets and Social Care Personal Budgets are severely circumscribed despite the legislative framework (Care Act 2014, operational from April 2015), which directs that all citizens who have *eligible social care needs* will have an entitlement to a personal budget. In addition, local authority eligibility thresholds are becoming increasingly tight and focused on meeting high-end (and, specifically, safeguarding) needs. In a statutory or local authority context, currently the only people eligible for social work intervention are, paradoxically, people with high-end health needs and adults with intellectual disabilities. The focus of these interventions, however, has traditionally been on the ways in which 'need' impacts upon a potential loss of 'independence'. That is, from a purely cynical perspective, how likely it will be that a person's needs will result in a local authority being required to fund long-term residential care. One of the ways, therefore, in which social work *has* responded to healthcare needs is to offset and delay dependence on the state. Thus, despite the medical imperative for social work support, the everyday ill body remains very much at the periphery of social work's professional attention.

In short, the political and policy context of social work, and its practice in local authority settings in the UK, means that social workers in this context have become managers of care packages and their associated bureaucracy. They are increasingly involved in setting, monitoring and achieving targets, and have little time left to build relationships with service users/clients and those people defined by the state as the most vulnerable. It is therefore unsurprising that the physical body and the daily experience of *chronic ill-health* fall largely outside the perceived purview of what constitutes vulnerability (or being at/presenting risk) and thus much of local authority (government sanctioned/funded) adult-related social work. The managerialist strategies that have become the key drivers of adult social work are, Twigg (2006: 121) suggests, non-corporeal in nature. Indeed, the tasks and practices associated with the body are seen to stand in sharp contrast to the quantifiable objectives of target driven, bureaucratically managed objectives (Saleeby, 1992).

The policy context of social work and social care is not one, we would suggest, which facilitates, notices and engages with the everyday lived experience of health and illness, particularly those autoimmune conditions, for example, that are seemingly (or are rendered) invisible. Rather, social work is increasingly in the business of managing resources for those labelled and assessed to be most at risk (or risky) and most vulnerable (Beddoe, 2014). Beddoe argues, 'within the current climate of the severe curtailment of welfare, the notion of vulnerability appears in the policy language to be connected by attempts by government to target funds, and thus programmes will focus on the most vulnerable who need to be protected' (Beddoe, 2014: 54). Furthermore, an emphasis on vulnerability and 'extremes of vulnerability' that drives access to social care services and social work management, can reduce a person's life to a series of risk factors, which does not adequately take account of experience (Fawcett, 2009: 474). As Fawcett (2009: 476) points out, emotional and human experiences that 'accompany bodily changes' are excluded in narrow constructions of vulnerability and procedural rationality that determines the identification of risk, vulnerability and the provision of care. The predetermined categories of vulnerability, therefore, with which social work operates and is most familiar, may well not embrace the 'bodily changes' and particular vulnerabilities experienced by people living with chronic conditions. This suggests two things. The first is that we need to look more closely at the place, role and value of social work in responding to the health and well-being of service users/clients in general, and those living with chronic ill-health in particular: and second, we need to be aware of the pitfalls, limitations and contradictions embedded in the notion of vulnerability. For not only does it potentially exclude a range of illness experience, is it one that is potentially paternalistic and stigmatising. Brown (2011: 319) suggests, 'like its conceptual cousin "risk", [vulnerability] has close links with choice, responsibility, blame and legitimacy' and should be 'handled with care'. Indeed, the political climate within which social workers currently operationalise the notion of vulnerability serves to further distance professionals from service users (and their healthy/unhealthy bodies). Operating at the furthest reaches of the notion, social workers engage most readily, as we have said, with those people perceived to be the most vulnerable and who thereby pose the greatest risk (to themselves and others). At the same time, contemporary policy, in the form of Direct Payments and the personalisation agenda, in placing responsibility for the management of both workers and finance firmly at the door of the individual service user (and their advocates and families), effectively displaces previously critical social work specific tasks. Social work is, then, thrust, in political, policy and personal contexts, out towards the margins of intervention. The corporeal realities of everyday life, the bodies, be they healthy or otherwise, of the people social work has traditionally engaged with are abstracted and 'disappeared' in the same ways in which the profession has been removed and displaced from direct, hands-on work with individuals and communities. An irony here, of course, is that, in recognising, and being at pains to actively take account of, myriad vulnerabilities and risks, the profession has, seemingly, neglected to either assess the quality of its own vulnerability or take cognisance of the very real risks to professional standing and credibility posed by the current political will.

If the ideological, legislative and organisational context is one possible explanation for the absence, and experience, of the physical body in social work, so too is the discipline's theoretical reluctance to engage with conceptualisations of corporeality. In part, Twigg (2006: 2) suggests that this may be due to (the dominance of) social policy's analytical approach to social care, where the focus, as we indicate above, is on institutional/rationalistic analysis, a tradition within which, 'new cultural analyses have made relatively little headway'. Tangenberg and Kemp (2002) similarly point to the lack of conceptual focus on the body in social work, despite the centrality of client bodies to everyday practice – it is the consequences of bodily actions (violence, addiction) that, instead, become the focus of theory and practice. Cameron and McDermott (2007) suggest that despite the fact that 'the person' has been placed at the centre of social work theory and practice, the human body has not received the same theoretical treatment: the focus has been 'all around' rather than centred on the body (person-centred but not body-centred) – it is, as we have noted, invisible, and taken for granted, in social work theory (and practice).

Social work has accorded biology a wide berth for reasons that, Saleeby (1992), Tangenberg and Kemp (2002) and Cameron and McDermott (2007) argue, are understandable. The profession, they suggest, has followed feminism in rejecting biological determinism. It has similarly, they claim, whole-heartedly rejected 'bad science' (eugenics), which has formed the basis of oppressive and discriminatory policy and practice. Moreover, social workers may be perceived to be reluctant to engage with a problem from a biological point of view in case this is 'medicalising' the issue and some social workers may be suspicious of positivist research methods, upon which biology is heavily reliant (Cameron and McDermott, 2007: 15; Giles, 2009). Social work's focus on 'social' and 'individual' (largely psychological) well-being, then, has been without any explicit consideration of the physical body. In conceptualising body work, Twigg et al. (2011: 175) similarly suggest that, even though the body would be considered 'central to the activities of health and social care, this fact is often obscured in accounts of the sector'. Status in professions, they argue, is denoted by distance *from* the body, so where doctors, for example, do engage in body work, the more demeaning aspects of it are bracketed off or referred to lesser status professions such as nursing; although one of the ways in which nursing has also sought to increase its professional status has been through a similar process of distancing and retreat. In other words, the further down the professional hierarchy, the 'messier' it gets and, thus, the less appealing both theoretically and in practice. In a similar vein, Twigg et al. (2011: 175) argue that 'social work in particular has traditionally defined its role as "not the body", handing over that territory to medicine', yet, paradoxically, social care is fundamentally *about* body care. As such, social work has, somewhat ironically, been at pains to distinguish itself from social care, which is regarded as unskilled, unqualified and 'dirty' work. In this way, social work has abrogated responsibility of both the 'scientific body' and the 'dirty body', thus further distancing the profession from the biological self. Social work deals on a daily basis with very messy aspects of humanity – 'soiled people' but not 'soiled bodies'. By relinquishing its position in undertaking and 'accounting for its undertaking' of body work to medicine and other health professionals (including occupational therapists and health visitors), social work has rendered the physical body invisible and, therefore, cannot incorporate within its professional remit, the everyday experiences of ill-health and the concomitant challenges to the promotion of well-being. On both accounts, the mundane bodily weariness of chronic, long-term, illness receives a double blow – not only are autoimmune conditions such as lupus experienced as 'invisible' and 'unseen', by both patients and clinicians, they seemingly don't belong to the work of the social work profession either. Paradoxically, then, person-centred, sociologically informed, anti-oppressive approaches to social work theory and practice (while a rejoinder to the biomedical master narrative), have effectively 'bleached out the corporeal' (Twigg et al., 2011: 175).

## Social work *is* health work

Here, with our aim being to re-conceptualise and reposition the body in the professional consciousness, we take as our starting point the conceptualisation of the body as both biological *and* social: the body has a 'material, biological base, that is altered and modified in social contexts' and is, as Nettleton and Watson (1998: 8) argue, socially contingent: 'how it is experienced will vary according to how, where and when it is located and the nature of the social relations which prevail'. This understanding is perhaps a necessary corrective to either taking the biological body for granted or dismissing its relevance, and we suggest that it is critical to relocate corporeality into the theory and practice of all dimensions of social work. If social work has not, as we have argued, been in the business of 'working with the physical body', it is unsurprising, therefore, that attention to the role and place of social work in addressing the body in health and illness, 'health work', is selective at best – an omission keenly felt by our clients/service users whose health, well-being and physical bodies are affected by their sometimes precarious social position, particularly those who are not regarded as most vulnerable or at risk.

McLeod and Bywaters (2000: 2) argued some 15 years ago that, 'In social work discourse in the UK, attention to physical health – never mind the consequences of practice for health inequalities – remains marginal, as it has been over the past thirty years', and similarly, Crisp and Beddoe (2013: 162) continue to demonstrate that health is very often an 'optional extra, an elective and rarely central to the social work curriculum'. Social work students may, therefore, continue to understand health and well-being to be outside of, or, at best, additional to, more 'immediate, critical tasks'. Yet, *all* social work is surely health work and *all* social work will have a health outcome, regardless of the field of intervention (substance use, child protection, fostering and adoption, bereavement, mental health, etc.). Physical health is an intrinsic part of being human and fundamentally shapes the quality of our lives. As we noted earlier, nowhere is the place of social work in the context of physical health more evident than in relation to health inequalities. Ill-health (and differential life expectancy that is acquired and compounded through limited life chances, poverty and isolation) is fundamentally unjust – an injustice that rests at the heart of the social work profession, the stated aim of which is to improve the lives of all people through reducing inequalities. Bywaters et al. (2009: 4) argue that social workers deal with the social determinants of ill health on a daily basis: 'it is hard to think of a social work contact in which damaged health is not already a factor or in which the issues under discussion will not influence future health'. Yet, social workers may not always be aware of, or focused on, the ways in which structural determinants might impact on the health of the people with whom they are working, compounded, of course, by the manner in which the physical body in social work (for all the reasons we identified above), is rendered invisible. The commonly held professional perception is that social work may only be involved in health work after illness that leads to specific and particular difficulties with daily living, or is specialist work that should take place in specialist settings.[1] This understanding, however, ignores the role that social work plays (or can play) in promoting good health in many other settings in which it operates (McLeod and Bywaters, 2000). We are, of course, also mindful of the structural difficulties practitioners already working in health settings may face in practice. Hospital social workers in the UK, for example, are under increasing pressure on a daily basis with quicker throughput of patients, extensive funding constraints, less accessible resources and the ever-changing and growing complexity of regulations and eligibility criteria and benefit delays; constraints that only serve to further remove specialist social work practice from health (and the body).

So, while social workers located within particular health settings, such as hospitals, hospices (in the context of palliative care social work) and some GP practices, have a particular role to play, it is clear that health work (body work) occurs across all social work settings. Bywaters et al. sum this up thus:

> Social work in all settings is concerned with the impact on people's lives of social forces which determine health chances and health experiences. Social workers, in all settings, are involved in processes which affect the health resources available to people – money, work, education and information, social and health services, networks and relationships, and emotional support – and their capacities to access and make use of them. Social workers in all settings need to integrate into their practice, awareness of the impact of poor health on people's everyday lives, their choices and opportunities.
>
> (Bywaters et al., 2009: 11)

Giles (2009) refers to this as a 'health equalities imagination', which requires that we not only pay attention to the physical body, but that we should be simultaneously cognisant of tackling health inequalities.

The Health and Social Care Act (2012) and the Care Act (2014) provide the current policy and legislative context within which social work with adults in the UK is located. One of the key thrusts of this legislation, whether it is reflected in the newly formed Clinical Commissions Groups or the Health and Wellbeing Boards, for example, is that local commissioners of health and social care and patient/user associations should work in an integrated way to support and improve local health and well-being (Department of Health, 2012). In this context, where health and social care are inextricably linked, it is ironic, if not unsurprising, that social work has never been more distant and separate from the professional practice of health work. Thus, the physical body, rather than becoming a central feature of social work theory and practice, is invisible and inaccessible, and our relationships with clients/service users ever more distant, perhaps 'personalised', but increasingly abstracted and individualised.

## The place of social work in chronic illness

Given our sense that social work has been legislatively and theoretically removed from the body (a shift in which the profession, as we note above, has been, perhaps unwittingly, complicit) our research on living with lupus offered an opportunity to explore respondents' experiences with social workers and whether they felt there might be a place for social work in living with and managing their illness. It is unsurprising, in the light of our arguments above, that no one we spoke with had met or worked with a social worker in the course of their illness.

**Victoria:** I've never come across a social worker, me.

**Andrew:** It was never offered, I've never even thought about it.

**Myf:** I don't think there is anything they can do for me.

There was little doubt, however, that respondents did identify a need for assessed support. Lucy was describing some of the mundane everyday challenges she faces and how wearing and demanding these can be:

> It's just stupid things you know. On some days it can be too painful to pick up the kettle and well just like opening a cap or something. You know I've had to call a neighbour across the road because I could not open the milk, you know, the cap, not because it was a new bottle or anything, it was just too painful, like today, this hand feels very swollen. I would appreciate help and will in the future, where someone will actually come to my home on a one-to-one basis and assess what your ability with lupus is and how debilitating it is and somebody to understand how to then be the go-between, between you and them, because it is distressing and stressful.

Lupus, for some people, is disruptive, unsettling and, on occasions, debilitating and life threatening – it can side-track, but not always derail, daily life (Miles, 2014). As with our study, the Ecuadorian women Miles (2014) writes of talk variously of lives where 'they occasionally feel tired, stiff, and sore while [for others] lupus has become a central, dominating motif of daily life as a life-threatening flare, seems to be looming [where] simple activities are often too much' (Miles, 2014: 12). Lupus and ambiguous chronic illness more generally, as we have suggested elsewhere, is a liminal experience (Stoller, 2004; Miles, 2014). This liminality, Miles (2014: 64) suggests 'is heavily oriented towards isolation and alienation and one that sees too little promise of future reincorporation into "normalcy"'. She continues, 'even when a lupus patient feels well… she knows she is different, susceptible, and vulnerable'. The uncertainty of lupus, of irregular bodily distress, in particular, poses significant challenges for social work, as it has, of course, for medicine and the process of diagnosis in particular. The respondent above very clearly articulates her stress and bodily distress. While acknowledging its shifting nature, she clearly articulates a need for acknowledgment and support while expressing anxiety about the future where her lupus may become more debilitating still. Social work needs to respond to a life lived with lupus when it is both side-tracked and derailed, chronic and life-threatening.

Respondents recognised, however, that help may only be forthcoming from social work (and social services more generally), in cases of 'extreme circumstances' despite the fact that the challenge of working positively with chronic illness lies most especially in the interstitial, liminal spaces that it occupies.

**Pamela:** I was thinking about this the other day actually, because I thought about my niece (who also has lupus), who is expecting a baby coming up to autumn, and she doesn't drive and I was thinking gosh, how is she going to cope, her husband's job is really busy. How is she going to cope with two tots in this condition? How is she going to get places? I know I've seen volunteer driving services in hospitals, but at the moment they seem to exist just for the elderly and people that are, you know, severely disabled.

The need for emotional and psychological support was also clearly identified.

**Andrew:** I think if a social worker can help patients with lupus or other illnesses, it's perhaps in terms of getting them to recognise that the illness is now part of them… it doesn't matter what you are doing, it isn't going to go away. It's important that you recognise that and live your life accordingly, because, I mean, you can't give up on life, that's just I think the worst thing you can possibly do, but if you recognise and accept it, then that gives you more ability to get on with it and cope with the things that it is throwing at you. Social workers are needed to help people mentally handle better what they are going through because there are an awful lot of people with lupus that don't really understand what's hit them… they just can't get their heads around it.

Navigating social services and accessing the appropriate benefit support, the traditional fayre of social work practice, was also clearly stressed. Gina described the difficulties she has had in this respect.

I was made to feel like a scrounger of this society, and I thought that was terrible, terrible because there isn't this understanding of this lupus illness, I mean I took it to [a fellow member of a lupus support group] and they took it to the MP and fought my corner fantastically but I am still under great scrutiny… you're fine, and then all your benefits stop and then you have to start all this again, you know, they were calling me every three months, every six months, but this last one [the member of the support group] came with me because I was having to go to appeal courts and it was horrible, I can't explain it to you, I've got a reprieve for now, you know, but the maximum is two years and I got the maximum but when that two years is up? It made me so ill, every day it was this anxiety going on, waiting for the letter, you know, was it accepted, wasn't it? Do I go for appeal? When is the appeal date, when is this, when is that? I literally would have needed a lawyer to help me cope with it, well I couldn't afford that so you have to get on with it and luckily I had [my friend in the support group] but what happens next time, you know, will they be able to help me?

Accessing and securing support from an opaque, ever-changing system of social work and care seemed to pose particular challenges for people with lupus, as it would for people living with similar shifting conditions and symptoms:

**Gina:** If you have got something seriously wrong with you, and you [hear], "sorry, all our benefits are reserved for other people"! It isn't right, and you know, lupus patients, because of the vagaries of the disease and the coming and going of it, you know, when, yeah, there are perhaps odd days when some of them are capable of working, but there are very few employers who will say come in when you feel well enough and stay at home when you don't. It doesn't happen that way in this world.

Mairs' (1990) essays on living with multiple sclerosis, talk most poignantly of what it means to live with a 'body in trouble'. A physical body in trouble stimulates and requires connections with self and others, including professionals – it is a catalyst for contact, a catalyst for acknowledging the biological. Tangenberg and Kemp (2002) suggest Mairs' experiences provide critical lessons for social workers. They point to the importance of physical well-being in the ways in which people make sense of their worlds and, as our respondents have said above, the impact of bodily troubles on daily life is profound – it is the minutiae, the seemingly irrelevant (the milk bottles, the car rides), which determine daily life lived with autoimmune conditions. Social workers therefore, have the professional responsibility to know and validate the lived experience of the body.

Living with a chronic illness (living with lupus) is taxing in every respect – physically, financially and emotionally (Miles, 2014) and the everyday lived experience of ambiguous chronic illnesses, such as lupus, is one of ongoing anxiety and daily bodily soreness. It is draining and demanding, reverberating throughout all aspects of life. Moreover, the invisibility and unpredictability of the illness brings its own bodily distress which 'bleeds into every other domain of life' (Miles, 2014: 12). Miles (2014) demonstrates how severe this bodily and emotional distress becomes in the context of poverty and social inequality. The precarious lives of the poor women in her study reflect narratives of struggle and loss – bodily, financial and material. Chronic illness, in this and other socio-economic contexts, thus interferes with social roles, status and functions. Drawing on Ware's (1999) work on the social course of chronic fatigue syndrome in the US, Miles (2014: 86) argues: 'Unable to participate fully in social life, the chronic illness sufferer finds herself increasingly marginalised at work and at home; her sense of identity becomes threatened as her ability to perform social [and economic] roles diminishes.' Chronic illness is thus exacerbated by poverty and inequality and becomes another marker and measure of marginality, yet, in the health and social care culture of extremes of risk and vulnerability, of working with thresholds that clearly preclude prevention, the effects of chronicity are often rendered invisible. The liminal, ambiguous space that chronic illness tends to occupy currently falls outside of social work's (and social care's) remit. The critical challenge for social work, therefore, is to make visible the invisible.

## Social work *is* body work

If chronic illness (and particularly ambiguous chronic illness) occupies a liminal space in the social work and social care agenda, then so too does the body. However, we argue here that social work *is* in the business of body work: corporeality *is* part and parcel of the everyday practice of social work. If social work lays claim to the body it can challenge the power of other professions to control the nature of social work practice and legitimately position its professional contribution at the very centre of health and social care (Lymbery, 2006). In this way, our engagement with health could be much more than selective and productive.

A number of social work scholars and practitioners are proposing ways in which social work can engage more effectively with 'the body'. Cameron and McDermott (2007), for example, suggest that social workers need to be 'body cognizant' and propose a Body Cognizant Assessment Guide to actively, if somewhat mechanically, place the body firmly into the process of social work assessment. This requires social workers to be aware of the impact of bio-psycho-socio-cultural-environmental factors on biological bodies. In a practice context, this means understanding the place and impact of our 'bodies' in social work interactions. In short, understanding 'the meanings ascribed by the worker, client and wider society to bodies and the significance of this to client well-being' (Cameron and McDermott, 2007: 87). Moreover, incorporating an understanding of 'corporeal capacity' as both a possible deficit and/or strength in our understanding of any social work interaction (those aversive as well as protective corporeal factors) further embed the biological body within social work's remit (Cameron and McDermott, 2007: 91). With a particular focus on health social work, Haultain (2014: 44–45) similarly points to a wide-ranging social work remit that incorporates cultural, emotional, medical and practical advocacy within the context of strong multidisciplinary teams in medical settings, in which social work's professional status is already effectively established. In another Australian study, exploring ways of improving psychosocial care for cancer patients in Melbourne, Lethborg and Posenelli (2009), outline an alternative way of working, where social workers were assigned to 'tumour/disease streams' rather than generic teams – the aim being to ensure a continuous relationship with each patient throughout their illness journey. Following the patient, and not simply the dictates of health service bureaucracy, is certainly a highly attractive approach, particularly in the context of lupus where the respondents in our study spoke of moving constantly between clinical departments, with little or no opportunity to piece together the jigsaw puzzle of their illness, or to voice the daily challenges of living with an ever shifting autoimmune condition.

The political and policy context of health and social care in the UK, which this situation reflects, continues to be in a state of flux, with recent legislative developments bringing about sweeping changes to the ways in which health and social care is commissioned and delivered (Health and Social Care Act, 2012; Care Act, 2014). These changes are taking place, as we have said, in the context of shrinking financial resources – both economically and ideologically impelled. While this places severe limitations on traditional social work practice in local authorities and hospitals (in respect of adults in need of support), it creates significant opportunities for development in other areas. The growing numbers of social enterprises in the UK (62,000 in 2011), for example, is testimony to this (King's Fund, 2011). The involvement of social work in the delivery of community-based, multidisciplinary health and social care is, of course, social work, but not as we might traditionally know it. Working within the framework of non-profit-making social and community enterprise may allow for more scope to engage, in ways we have advocated, the invisible 'chronically ill' body, for, within this context, recognition of the social determinants of health and disease are central. Marmot Review (2010) and the recent World Health Organization

(2014) European review on the Social Determinants of Health identify six themes to improve health outcomes and reduce inequalities: a human rights approach based on citizenship; building resilience of individuals and communities; the importance of every stage of the life course; protection of future generations from social and economic inequalities; systematic, scaled, collaborative action; and a proportionate universalist approach. In these contexts, individual (and family) control over illness is central to building resilience: this is arguably critical (and most certainly missing) in the context of many autoimmune conditions. The opportunity to generate control and recognise, if not alleviate, the everyday challenges of chronicity, is one that social work, with other professionals, should not miss.

(Ambiguous) chronic illness has been invisible to social work, yet, we have argued, the body, and concomitantly its health, is at the very centre of social work practice and, as such, it is the bodily knowing and physical experiences of everyday life that need to take centre-stage. As such, we would advocate for a return to some of social work's fundamental, underpinning values, practices and principals; those that have concrete foundations in the interpersonal relationships we have traditionally shared with those we work with (specifically, those relationships side-lined and, arguably, discarded, in the flotsam and jetsam of strategic/political change). This demands a cognisance, and foregrounding, of the relationship that sits at the very heart of social work practice – that which is grounded in traditional equalities based social work, a space where the social and biological body can be effectively united and aligned. The biological body must, therefore, be placed alongside the social body in reasserting the responsibility of social work for 'body work'. In this way, the profession can, perhaps, begin to address the invisibility to which we have referred.

## Notes

1  There are a number of voluntary organisations/charities that employ social workers in specialist health contexts, such as the Multiple Sclerosis Society.

## References

Beddoe, L. (2014) 'Risk and Vulnerability Discourses in Health'. In L. Beddoe and J. Maidment (eds), *Social Work Practice for Promoting Health and Well being: Critical Issues*. Oxford: Routledge.

British Academy (2014) *'If You Could Do One Thing…' Nine Local Actions to Reduce Health Inequalities*. London: British Academy.

Brown, K. (2011) '"Vulnerability": Handle with Care'. *Ethics and Social Welfare* 5(3): 313–321.

Bywaters, P., McLeod, E. and Napier, L. (2009) 'Social Work and Global Health Inequalities'. In P. Bywaters, E. McLeod and L. Napier (eds), *Social Work and Global Health Inequalities: Practice and Policy Developments*. Bristol: Policy Press.

Cameron, N. and McDermott, F. (2007) *Social Work & the Body*. Basingstoke: Palgrave Macmillan.

Care Act 2014, www.legislation.gov.uk/ukpga/2014/23/contents/enacted (accessed 8 September 2014).

Community Care Act (Direct Payments) Act 1996. London: HMSO.

Crisp, B. R. and Beddow, L. (2013) 'Conclusion: Developing an Agenda to Promote Health and Well-being in Social Work Education'. In, B. R. Crisp and L. Beddoe (eds), *Promoting Health and Well-being in Social Work Education*. London: Routledge.

Department of Health (2005) *Supporting People with Long Term Conditions: An NHS and Social Care Model to Support Local Innovation and Integration.* London: HMSO.

Department of Health (2008) *Your Health, Your Way: A Guide to Long-Term Conditions and Self Care.* London: Department of Health.

Department of Health (2010) *Equity and Excellence: Liberating the NHS.* London: Department of Health.

Department of Health (2012) *Long-Term Conditions Compendium of Information,* www.gov.uk/government/uploads/system/uploads/attachment_data/file/216528/dh_134486.pdf (accessed 2 August 2014).

Dominelli, L. (1996) 'Deprofessionalising Social Work: Anti-Oppressive Practice, Competencies and Postmodernism'. *British Journal of Social Work* 26: 153–175.

Fawcett, B. (2009) 'Vulnerability: Questioning the Certainties in Social Work and Health'. *International Social Work* 52(4): 473–484.

Ferguson, I. (2007) 'Increasing User Choice or Privatising Risk? The Antinomies of Personalisation'. *British Journal of Social Work* 37: 387–403.

Foster, A. and Roberts, V. Z. (1999) *Managing Mental Health in the Community: Chaos and Containment.* London: Routledge.

Giles, R. (2009) 'Developing a Health Equality Imagination: Hospital Practice Challenges for Social Work Priorities'. *International Social Work* 52(4): 525–537.

Glenndinning, C., Halliwell, S., Jacobs, S., Rummery, K. and Tyler, J. (2000) *Bridging Independence: Using Direct Payments to Integrate Health and Social Services.* Bristol: Policy Press.

Harlow, E. (2003) 'New Managerialism, Social Service Departments and Social Work Practice Today'. *Practice* 15(2): 29–44.

Harlow, E., Berg, E., Barry, J. and Chandler, J. (2013) 'Neoliberalism, Managerialism and the Reconfiguration of Social Work in Sweden and the United Kingdom'. *Organisation* 20(4): 534–550.

Haultain, L. (2014) 'Facing the Challenges Together: A Future Vision for Health Social Work'. In, L. Beddoe and J. Maidment (eds), *Social Work Practice for Promoting Health and Well being: Critical Issues.* Oxford: Routledge.

Health and Social Care Act 2012, www.legislation.gov.uk/ukpga/2012/7/pdfs/ukpga_20120007_en.pdf (accessed 8 September 2014).

Institute of Health Equity (2014) *Marmot Indicators 2014: A Preliminary Summary with Graphs,* www.instituteofhealthequity.org/projects/marmot-indicators-2014 (accessed 15 October 2014).

Killaspy, H. (2006) 'From the Asylum to Community Care: Learning from Experience'. *British Medical Bulletin* 1(79–80): 245–258.

King's Fund (2011) *Social Enterprise in Health Care: Promoting Organisation Autonomy and Staff Engagement.* London: King's Fund.

Lethborg, C. and Posenelli, S. (2009) 'Improving Psychosocial Care for Cancer Patients'. In P. Bywaters, E. McLeod and L. Napier (eds), *Social Work and Global Health Inequalities: Practice and Policy Developments.* Bristol: Policy Press.

Lymbery, M. (2001) 'Social Work at the Crossroads'. *British Journal of Social Work* 31: 369–384.

Lymbery, M. (2006) 'United We Stand? Partnership Working in Health and Social Care and the Role of Social Work in Services for Older People'. *British Journal of Social Work* 36: 1119–1134.

Lymbery, M. (2012) 'Social Work and Personalisation'. *British Journal of Social Work* 42: 783–792.

Mairs, N. (1990) *Carnal Acts.* New York: HarperCollins.

Marmot Review (2010) *Fair Society. Healthy Lives*, www.instituteofhealthequity.org/projects/fair-society-healthy-lives-the-marmot-review (accessed 15 October 2014).

McLaughlin, H. (2009) 'What's in a Name? "Client", "Patient", "Customer", "Consumer", "Expert by Experience", "Service User" – What's Next?' *British Journal of Social Work* 39: 1101–1117.

McLeod, E. and Bywaters, P. (2000) *Social Work, Health and Equality*. London: Routledge.

Miles, A. (2014) *Living with Lupus: Women and Chronic Illness in Ecuador*. Austin: University of Texas Press.

National Health Service and Community Care Act 1990, www.legislation.gov.uk/ukpga/1990/19/contents (accessed 8 September 2014).

Nettleton, S. and Watson, J. (1998) 'The Body in Everyday Life: An Introduction'. In S. Nettleton and J. Watson (eds), *The Body in Everyday Life*. London: Routledge.

Postle, K. (2001) 'The Social Work Side is Disappearing: I Guess it Started with us being Called Care Managers'. *Practice* 13(1): 13–26.

Saleeby, D. (1992) 'Biology's Challenge to Social Work: Embodying the Person-in-environment Perspective'. *Social Work* 37: 112–118.

Sanderson, T., Calnan, M., Morris, M., Richards, P. and Hewlett, S. (2011) 'Shifting Normalities: Interactions of Changing Conceptions of a Normal Life and the Normalisation of Symptoms in Rheumatoid Arthritis'. *Sociology of Health & Illness* 33(4): 618–633.

Stoller, P. (2004) *Stranger in the Village of the Sick: A Memoir of Cancer, Sorcery, and Healing*. Boston: Beacon Press.

Tangenberg, K. and Kemp, S. (2002) 'Embodied Practice: Claiming the Body's Experience, Agency and Knowledge for Social Work'. *Social Work* 47(1): 9–18.

Twigg, J. (2006) *The Body in Health and Social Care*. Basingstoke: Palgrave Macmillan.

Twigg, J., Wolkowitz, C., Cohen, R. L. and Nettleton, S. (2011) 'Conceptualising Body Work in Health and Social Care'. *Sociology of Health and Illness* 33(2): 171–188.

Ware, N. (1999) 'Toward a Model of Social Course in Chronic Illness: The Example of Chronic Fatigue Syndrome'. *Culture, Medicine and Psychiatry* 23(3): 303–331.

World Health Organization (2014) *Review of Social Determinants and the Health Divide in the WHO European Region Update*. Denmark: WHO.

# Conclusion

We began this book in a beige waiting room in an NHS rheumatology clinic and it makes sense, in conclusion, to return to this space that has become, for ourselves and the people who participated in some of the research we draw on in this text, a common and constant theme in our lives. It has come to represent the complexity, frustrations and many battles long-term illness has presented.

In the course of writing the book, our illnesses have continued to be woven into the fabric of our lives, constituting a binding thread that inextricably links our own lives to those of the people we write about. We have witnessed, and have been part of, the many battles, triumphs and losses people have experienced while living with autoimmunity and our own illnesses have permitted us a very particular insight into the experience of living with an illness without cure. For us both, the waiting room has acquired a growing significance. For one, this has meant an unstable and shifting experience as the shape of illness, including the original diagnosis, has changed over time, suspected lupus becoming limited systemic sclerosis (scleroderma). It has also come to include the diagnosis of an additional long-term condition (adrenal insufficiency), which only serves to further complicate the illness experience – living with co-morbidities is, thus, now a personal, as well as a theoretical experience. For the other, gradual deterioration of the joints and disfigurement (which is keenly felt and increasingly publicly evident) and the prospect of more intrusive immunosuppressants is a daily feature of life with rheumatoid arthritis. Despite the challenges faced on a daily basis, for us both, however, we engage productively in, and with, the world that, for the most part, remains unaware of the fact or impact of illness, which is largely unseen and unacknowledged. The severity of illness, of course, will determine the extent to which illness intrudes and disrupts 'normal' life, but our biographical work continues nonetheless.

We would venture that our experience of illness, in all its forms, may be similar for many people living with autoimmunity, yet, this increasingly ubiquitous illness experience is often hidden and the voice of those who live with autoimmunity is relatively silent (a silence that is evident in the fact that it is only by way of a US television drama, *House*, that lupus has acquired a popular and public resonance). We were particularly struck at a very early stage of this research by the challenges that diagnosis presented – people's stories were replete with years of diagnostic struggle and despair largely, we would suggest, because the diagnostic possibility of autoimmunity does not easily occur in the clinic, particularly in the context of diffuse and wide-ranging symptoms that conditions such as lupus present. Inadvertently, perhaps, it thus became clear that, in giving voice to our respondents, we were also giving voice to the silence of autoimmunity.

In considering the nature and extent of this silence, we simultaneously came to explore and understand the professional responses to autoimmunity. While sometimes literally life-saving, these responses are processed and ordered both by the bureaucracy of the health service and the disciplinary divisions of labour that tend to shape and fracture clinical practice. These fractures are particularly striking in the context of lupus, a condition that highlights and underpins the uncertainties and underlying unequal power relationships embedded in the contemporary clinical encounter. In the context of our own professional practice, the silence of auto-immunity, and indeed the ill body more generally, is particularly profound. We had anticipated some degree of absence in the context of social work, what we had not expected was the deafening silence that actually pertains for both patients and practitioners alike.

How then, do we begin to give meaning to, and generate awareness of, the physical body and the ill body in social work and, further, how do we reconcile and address the absences in the professional understanding and response to autoimmunity that we have highlighted? In short, what do the concepts and issues we have raised mean for the process and practice of contemporary social work?

As we have demonstrated, a biomedical tradition and a particular policy context in health and social care have come together to effectively obfuscate the 'social' from social work. This has generated a cohort of practitioners, in the UK at least, who are obligated to practice in ways that may be described as lacking a social cognisance of the body. That is, as social workers, we are familiar with brokering the body, and assisting service users to manage their own bodies, yet this is quite often at the cost of an understanding of those very physical bodies in the social environments and social relationships within which they operate. In this context, it is something of an irony that the current legislation that fundamentally shapes our work with adult service users (Health and Social Care Act, 2012; Care Act, 2014), effectively oversees and promotes the absence of the social (and relationship led social work) to which we refer.

In order to explore and address these issues, we need to think, first, about what we understand social work to be. If it is to remain a largely body-blind profession, then little is to be gained from this exploration. We would argue, however, that there is a critical space for social work's particular value base and professional perspective in the world of autoimmunity and in the clinics that diagnose, treat and manage these most enigmatic of conditions. This, however, requires a body cognisant (Cameron and McDermott, 2007) social worker, one who is able to purposefully 'think body' in the midst of everyday practice situations. For, in the context of contemporary disease experiences, the ill body is often to be found in the most unanticipated places. As such, the origins and effects of autoimmunity need to be sought out, as the hidden nature of these conditions can, as we have demonstrated, make them opaque and difficult to discern.

To think differently about social work in this context means to understand its value and application beyond the purview of the limitations of traditional and policy-led definitions of vulnerability and intervention. There is, perhaps, a general consensus that 'proper social work' is to be found in certain agencies and locations and among certain groups of people, namely those legally defined at 'risk' at either end of the life-course; those who by virtue of disability are also deemed to be at risk and, of course, those who might present a risk either to themselves or others. We would argue for an extension to this limiting remit – an invocation of 'social work, but not as we know it'. In the context of social work and autoimmunity, then, social work could happen in places where you might not expect it, with people who may not traditionally be regarded as a/at risk and who are 'vulnerable' in ways that defy (and underpin) current policy and practice. Vulnerability, then, is both an experience and a consequence that can apply to any of us. It is not a notion that is exclusive to those deemed thus by shifts in policy or practice.

At present, social work is perceived to be most active, and effective, in the protection of young people and adults, when, as we have argued, vulnerability and its effects are to be felt and enacted in far wider, and sometimes unexpected, contexts. The disease conditions of which we write in this book (lupus, rheumatoid arthritis, multiple sclerosis, etc.) are not simply the preserve of 'vulnerable' children or adults. Rather, while demographic evidence suggests that they are clearly gendered and, in some cases, racialised, these conditions are most often those that affect people in their most productive and, arguably, resilient years. This is not to say, of course, that existing vulnerability (socio-economic vulnerability in particular) is not profoundly exacerbated by the onset of physical illness.

While social workers already enjoy professional responsibilities unavailable to other professions (the statutory capacity to intervene, for example) we also need to think about how the particularities of the social work role can be brought to bear in more enabling contexts, bringing what we would argue is a unique, anti-oppressive, progressive value base to interactions with the ill body that might be of particular value to people with ongoing ill-health, particularly autoimmune conditions. This, of course, requires a new understanding of the place and value of social work, not just from within the profession itself. If the body and ill-health are largely invisible in social work, the social work profession is completely absent in the lexicon of many clinicians – medicine and nursing in particular. It is not surprising, therefore, to find the views and perspectives of social work are difficult to assert and enact in clinical situations where people living with long-term illness may find themselves. We would argue that social work has a justified place in clinical medical practice, not simply one that provides a lone voice on, for example, the vagaries of the benefit system, but is integral to the impacts and effects of the diagnosis, treatment and management of bodily pain, illness and distress.

There could be, we would argue, a specific place for social work in the rheumatology clinic (the clinical home of autoimmune conditions), in particular, where the social worker might provide a critical link between multiple patient needs while enabling medical practitioners to make connections between disparate symptoms and experiences – drawing together, for both patient and practitioner, the pieces of the patchwork. We would advocate for a professional who 'follows the patient's symptoms' between multiple clinical specialisms, accompanying the person on an autoimmune journey that is undertaken from the vantage point of an explicit understanding of the autoimmune body. In practice, this would mean assisting the patient to navigate the various waypoints on the journey.

By way of example, as we highlighted in the previous chapter, Lethborg and Posenelli (2009: 201) suggest a model of practice, in the context of a cancer social work team, whereby social workers were assigned to 'tumour streams rather than treatment units in order to ensure a continuous relationship with each patient throughout their journey. The model also aimed to provide earlier intervention and assistance in navigating the hospital system, regardless of the availability of streamed clinical care pathways.' Professionals, therefore, follow the patient, providing a personalised service that helps to reduce the atomised type of experiences more traditional hospital models would generate, while also providing psychosocial support, reducing a person's isolation and the amount of work they are required to undertake to navigate the patchwork of contemporary medicine that is so clearly reflected in the many clinical divisions in the hospital setting. We would caution, however, against a literal interpretation of this model that situates the social worker, in the context of physical illness, only in the clinical context, for we would wish to reiterate our central point that *all* social work is body work and *all* social work is health work. It is not possible to sidestep or be blind to the embodied realities of ill-health in any context.

So where does an awareness of the possibilities of a body-cognisant social work begin? As social work educators, we would advocate for a reinvigoration of social work training that refocuses the professional consciousness on an holistic reading of the human condition (something that, perhaps, has been lost in the increasing specialisation and partitioning of social work provision, much like the clinical medical practice we describe earlier). The contemporary political and policy imperative to 'carve up' social work into its constituent service user silos, with the attendant professional myopia that results, explicitly invites a disaggregation of the body and its physical and social meanings. Embedding this awareness into the initial qualifying training of social workers would, of course, require us to revisit the central aims and objectives of professional training.

What we would purposefully refute in this context is that this suggestion provides a rationale for a backward-looking or reductionist approach to the body and its place in social work. Rather, what we are suggesting, is that providing a critical space for the body (both social and physical) in professional social work practice, allows for a more purposefully discursive understanding of what is means to be 'vulnerable' and 'at risk'. As Cameron and McDermott (2007: 4) suggest, in the various contexts within which social workers operate – in health and illness, child welfare, housing, community development, with those who experience mental distress or disabilities, end of life care and the various safeguarding arenas – in the practical and existential realties of day to day practice 'how the body is afflicted, treated, cared for, supported and nurtured is of primary concern… placing the body at the centre of theorising and practice is vital to social work's espoused mission and purpose'.

The biographical work that we, the patients we have spoken with, and the practitioners who support us, have undertaken, whether through the use of immunosuppressants or social repair and support (with or without the help of a social worker), suggests that we are all engaged in the same pursuit – that of continual biographical development and restitution. Yet, the conundrum we all face is the autoimmune paradox – the challenge of having to literally manage the self (living with a biological insurgent in residence) in ways which other conditions do not demand. The question 'do I hate myself because my body is destroying itself?', asked of us by a colleague diagnosed with an autoimmune condition, is one that people living with other conditions are not impelled to ask or answer and it lies, as we have said, at the very heart of the autoimmune experience. This person framed this paradox by placing it within a lexicon of other potentially self-destructive behaviours, saying 'fairly soon after I was diagnosed, when a lot was going on, in many ways I felt I did do quite a lot of self-destruction. I just wondered if the body attacking itself was in some sense metaphoric'.

Whether metaphoric or not, manipulation of the self is how we are forced to manage our conditions, but these are the types of disease that we are never really going to resolve. So, while we engage in a range of competing forms of biographical work, all in an effort to contain and suppress the aberrant self (which many people will never have perceived to be misbehaving), this will always be an ongoing battle (biomedical and social) that characterises the very particular experience of living with autoimmunity.

In conclusion, then, it is the autoimmune paradox that has constituted one of the central and most critical threads throughout our work. We have woven this notion into a dialogue between different and often divergent disciplinary traditions (for example, social work and digital sociology, and social work and medicine), exploring lupus as an autoimmune experience, not only an example of a long-term condition. In doing so, we have simultaneously generated a potential conversation within the social work profession that might focus more explicitly and purposefully on the place of the ill body in the professional consciousness. Our hope is that this will foreground the autoimmune experience while creating a place for social work in the hugely complex journey those experiencing autoimmunity undertake.

## References

Cameron, N. and McDermott, F. (2007) *Social Work & the Body*. Basingstoke: Palgrave Macmillan.

Care Act 2014, www.legislation.gov.uk/ukpga/2014/23/contents/enacted (accessed 8 September 2014).

Health and Social Care Act 2012, www.legislation.gov.uk/ukpga/2012/7/pdfs/ukpga_2012 0007_en.pdf (accessed 9 April 2015).

Lethborg, C. and Posenelli, S. (2009) 'Improving Psychosocial Care for Cancer Patients'. In P. Bywaters, E. McCleod and L. Napier (eds), *Social Work and Global Health Inequalities. Practice and Policy Developments*. Bristol: Policy Press.

# Appendix

## Notes on research methodology

The original research we refer to throughout this book derives from a wider study entitled 'Transitions to Illness: The Lived Experience of Systemic Lupus Erythematosus'. Data collection was undertaken between July 2010 and February 2013. The central research question our study asked was: How do people with lupus understand, experience and live their illness? It explored the following six themes:

- The process of 'becoming ill', specifically, how living with an autoimmune condition such as lupus impacts upon a person's sense of self and identity.
- The nature and experience of people's encounters with members of the medical profession, including GPs, consultants and specialist nurses.
- How lupus influences family/intimate relationships and people's experiences of giving and receiving care.
- The ways in which people accommodate lupus in their everyday lives.
- The role of support networks (both virtual and organisational) in shaping the illness experience.
- The place of the (ill) body and 'body work' in social work.

The study, funded by both Lupus UK and the University of Hull Faculty Strategic Support Fund, was granted approval by the relevant University Ethics Committee.

In conducting the research, we utilised a qualitative research design and drew on a range of qualitative research methods including focus groups, narrative interviews, artistic representations of illness and a research blog. The blog has become a popular contemporary medium through which both the experience and discourse of chronic illness and disease are played out. The internet is saturated with self-help fora, blogs and personal homepages that offer unique possibilities for individuals whose engagement in collective discussion and opportunities for delivering personal discourse in the 'real world' may be limited by physical, and/or psychological factors. In the same way that the online environment provides people, with a similar diagnosis, the opportunity to share their illness experiences, our research blog served to provided a dedicated space for participants (in the UK) to explore and share their experience of living with lupus. Respondents were informed of the purpose of the blog and that we were administering and running it. The blog's front page can be accessed at http://transitionstoillness.blogspot.co.uk. Respondents were recruited through other relevant internet fora, such as Facebook and the Lupus UK website, although the blog was publicly available, so, in theory, it could have been accessed by anyone.

The blog initially ran for a period of three months and we (both registered social workers) managed it daily, responding to contributors' comments within 24 hours, thus encouraging active participation. Discussion on the blog was guided by the use of specific 'threads', for example: What were your first symptoms and experiences of the illness? Other threads explored the transition to an illness identity and the effects of illness on relationships. The number of contributors to the blog was between 40 and 45 (some contributors chose to use pseudonyms and some anonymous contributors posted more than once, though seldom more than three times in any one thread). The blog generated 148 separate posts (a total of 264 including researchers' responses). After an initial three-month period, the data generated through the blog were analysed and informed the further three phases of research. The blog has also functioned as a vehicle through which we have kept contributors up-to-date with the progress of the research and it was also a forum in which to ask if contributors would be willing to be involved in other aspects of the work. The research blog, unexpectedly, came to adopt and mirror many of the characteristics of online support groups as discussed in Chapter 6.

We are aware of the challenges online research can present, including (ironically in the context of our discussions throughout this book on the search for legitimacy through diagnosis), issues of integrity and authenticity. Yet, online research has become an integral part of the lexicon of data collection techniques and methods (Kozinets, 2010; Salmons, 2010). As noted above, some contributors, although very few, chose to use pseudonyms for posting on threads and were, therefore, not available to speak to or communicate with outside of the intimate space of the 'blogosphere'. Other contributors agreed to follow-up e-mails and/or interviews. 'Blog respondents' were, therefore, wholly self-selected and also clearly represent a particular cohort of people familiar and comfortable with engagement in an online context. We are also aware that the online environment constitutes something of a demographically and socially mediated (by, for example, age and/or ability) landscape. Moreover, those whose diagnosis, and subsequent experience of lupus, was relatively straightforward and/or swift would be less likely to access the blog.

Following the completion of the research blog we interviewed a total of 30 people across the UK. This number includes a focus group in the north-west of England, convened by members of the north-west branch of Lupus UK. The use of multiple (and mixed) methods of data collection allowed for the triangulation of data.

Face-to-face interviews were conducted in a traditional semi-structured format. With the exception of three interviews, all were conducted by both researchers. With the permission of the interviewees, all interviews were recorded and transcribed verbatim. Analysis of the data was conducted using a modified grounded theory approach. On the blog, as each thread developed, material was codified and thematised. The blog constituted what might be termed a textual conversation that allowed for a reading and analysis of the respondents' narratives as they occurred. Both researchers read and analysed data from the blog and clarified emerging themes as they arose. This permitted both dual researcher analysis and inter-researcher reliability. Interview and focus group data were similarly managed – coding and thematising was under-taken simultaneously. The identity of the respondents quoted in the text of the book have been protected with the use of pseudonyms. We have accorded the same sig-nificance to all sources of empirical evidence presented in the book (blog, interviews, focus groups and art work).

## References

Kozinets, R. V. (2010) *Nenography: Doing Ethnographic Research Online*. London: Sage Publications.

Salmons, J. E. (2010) *Online Interviews in Real Time*. London: Sage Publications.

# Index

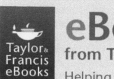